READING MENTAL HEALTH NURSING
EDUCATION, RESEARCH & POWER

Lanchester Library

WITHDRAWN

LANCHESTER LIBRARY, Coventry University

Gosford Street, Coventry, CV1 5DD Telephone 024 7688 7555

ONE WEEK LOAN COLLECTION

This book is due to be returned not later than the date and time stamped above. Fines are charged on overdue books

For Elsevier:
Commissioning Editor: Steven Black
Development Editor: Fiona Conn
Project Manager: Kerrie-Anne Jarvis
Designer: George Ajayi

READING MENTAL HEALTH NURSING: EDUCATION, RESEARCH, ETHNICITY & POWER

Liam Clarke
RN DipEd DipTheol DipMedPhil BA MSc MA PhD
Reader in Mental Health, University of Brighton, Eastbourne, UK

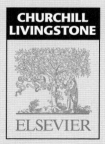

CHURCHILL LIVINGSTONE

ELSEVIER

Edinburgh London New York Oxford Philadelphia
St Louis Sydney Toronto 2008

CHURCHILL
LIVINGSTONE
ELSEVIER

An imprint of Elsevier Limited

First published 2008

ISBN: 978-0-443-10384-1

British Library Cataloguing in Publication Data
A catalogue record for this book is available from the British Library

Library of Congress Cataloging in Publication Data
A catalog record for this book is available from the Library of Congress

Notice
Neither the Publisher nor the author assumes any responsibility for any loss or injury and/or damage to persons or property arising out of or related to any use of the material contained in this book. It is the responsibility of the treating practitioner, relying on independent expertise and knowledge of the patient, to determine the best treatment and method of application for the patient.

The Publisher

Working together to grow
libraries in developing countries
www.elsevier.com | www.bookaid.org | www.sabre.org

 ELSEVIER   BOOK AID International   Sabre Foundation

Printed in China

Dedication

For Myra Bonella (nee O'Driscoll)

Contents

Foreword

Knowingness can be very seductive, it can make us feel powerful, less anxious, just plain right. And it is so much less tiring than not knowing as anyone who has ever tried to learn Mandarin, the Saxophone or Algebra will tell you. Staying enchanted and curious is hard. Being surefooted and knowing is easier to bear. But not necessarily right.

Arguably, when mental health nursing moved into the universities there was something of a rush toward 'knowing'. Let's face it there had to be: many mental health lecturers carried around this vague paranoia that the real academics, the dusty men with hair in their ears over in Physics, Economics and quite surprisingly the new Performance Arts Department, were smirking at them from behind their doctorates. Staying curious and uncertain can be difficult enough without a load of pompous people looking at you and thinking you might be stupid because you're a nurse.

But nursing is nothing if not adaptable and adapt it did. It became a social science of sorts. A discipline of its time: self-referential and preoccupied with method. If people are going to spend money on health care, so the argument goes, we want to know absolutely that we are buying care that works. And if you want to know, really know in this era, you ask Dr. Science.

And that's fine. We like Dr. Science, we've seen his work in cancer care, fertility treatment, and heart disease and we know he can be an incredible force for good. And it made sense, given the pressure we were under to quickly establish a method or knowledge base or intellectual paradigm to import him into mental health academia and begin to build. Of course it isn't quite the same, the drugs don't work quite as well and nobody has yet come up with a way of opening up someone's head and removing the depression although I'm sure its just a matter of time before they try, but hey, its better then guessing, right? Or Homeopathy.

But is Dr Science enough? Far be it from me to suggest you watch really good Kung Fu films but I can't help thinking Bruce Lee had a point when he says to an over-anxious student at the beginning of *Enter the Dragon*: 'It is like a finger pointing away to the moon, don't concentrate on the finger or we will miss all that heavenly glory.' In mental health we spend an awful lot of time staring at the finger, albeit often as part of a randomized controlled trial.

The reality of mental health care is that our attempts to understand it as part of the human condition can be informed by so much more than social science. Granted Philosophy, History, Economics, Literature and Film Studies are less likely to offer us the temporary truths that sociology claims to provide but they can inform our understanding and they can help us to think critically about the world in which we live, the power relations we construct and most important, the underpinning morality of what we are engaged in.

We can't afford to abandon mature thought. We can't be so arrogant as to imagine that Plato, Descartes, Marx, Foucault or even Thomas Szasz can't help inform the way we construct ourselves as human beings living together, or indeed our understanding of what mental health difficulty might be. It is the responsibility of the curious to ask questions: in mental health care it is the responsibility of academics, teachers, service providers and professionals to carry those questions sometimes unanswered because that is what intelligent and responsible people sometimes have to do. To stay curious, to look beyond the obvious and to broaden the criteria we have for the truth.

But of course our responsibilities go beyond asking good questions and reading interesting books. Without some kind of moral position, without a commitment to something of value, the capacity to love or at least care about something, critical thinking – any kind of thinking – is essentially just bar talk. A vanity for the disengaged. It is the drive to think carefully, systematically and with purpose that makes critical thinking a thing of value.

Mental health care: the activity, the reams of policy, the human exchange needs all the thinking it can get. If we can borrow ways of understanding the world from historians or philosophers or even, God forbid, economists, and those ideas enhance understanding or empower patients or carers then let's borrow. At a time when motifs like 'evidence-based practice' seek to limit the way we think about the health issues we care about, it is, it seems to me, pretty timely that we try to look beyond demonstrable or fundable theory and toward informed and relentless inquiry.

And that is what this book tries to do: it inquires, with a notable academic rigor and with an inventiveness that is too rare in mental health writing. It is a skilled and well-thought out attempt to look at the world in which we work and develop our understanding in a way that may have professional benefit and moral purpose. And it is informed not by the counting sciences but rather by philosophy, history, literature and sociology, disciplines that in the view of some people at least, mirror the fluidity of mental health care. Are you going to agree with the author? Who knows, but therein lies the key. It is not our responsibility always to be right, no matter what we do; it is our responsibility to stay curious and to pursue good.

Mark Radcliffe
Southampton 2007

Preface

We are now in an age of biological psychiatry, a psychiatry which sees as embarrassing any psychology that chooses to ignore tangible indices of effectiveness, the so-called 'evidence base'.

There is nothing wrong with evidence, of course, except when the testimony of individuals is ruled inadmissible as such. In light of this, it is timely to ask if psychiatric nurses seek to embrace an approach that combines biology with behaviourism or, alternatively, continue with a post-Enlightenment tradition which allows mental distress its hinterlands of economy, history, religion, culture and ethnicity.

Constructing orthodoxies entails belittling one's opponents; hence, questions of how psychiatric nursing might progress are contestations about power. For instance, we need to distrust an anti-intellectualism that would limit nursing practice to measurable determinants and which reduces distinctions between science and talking about science. Indeed, the proselytising of science by some psychiatric nurses has acquired dogmatic proportions.

This book's origins lie in an interview with the philosopher Sir Frederick Ayer. Insisting that language only values what can be empirically verified, Sir Freddy was asked what evidence he would seek were his wife to assert the proposition 'I love you'. Now, many disappointed lovers have learned the hard way that saying 'I love you' may conceal duplicitous intentions. However, that surely is the point: that much communication lies outside testable fields, that interplays of language and 'being with' are important elements of humanity and thus of the psychiatric nurse's role. A too-easy adoption of outcome-based therapies, of nurse prescribing and so forth may emasculate whatever the essence of psychiatric nursing might be. There cannot prevail an evidence base – of the empirical kind desired by Sir Frederick Ayer – because love, justice and ethics are as relevant to our self-evident human nature as anything else. Equally, however, we need to avoid an existential imperialism that denies categories of mental disorder altogether and, particularly, that faddish post-modernism that perpetually self-celebrates its intolerance of the possibility of truth.

This is a declarative and explorative text. Some ideas readers will disagree with, the more so because this is not a 'seeing both sides of the question' text. I doubt there are, necessarily, other sides. Rather do I set out a 'stall of interests' whose inherent problems incite no easy answers and which may even prove off-putting to some.

Liam Clarke
Eastbourne 2007

Introduction

This book is about power – its possession by some, non-possession by others, its situation within language, imagery, organisations, roles, rituals, ethnicities, professions, imagination. Power is identity; the more one accounts for one's identity in relation, the more one influences the scheme of things, claims one's territory, defines it, defends it, extends it, celebrates it, publishes it, relinquishes it. Medicine is the primary case in point: a profession of mythic proportions in the West, its status proportionate to its intimacy with life and death. Not that its persona hasn't slipped of late; the demand for evidence-based practice has had a levelling effect, as has rising consumerism and the 'informed patient'. But more so have scarcer facilities, and educational expansion, exerted a determining impact: the hothouse economics of health provision have accelerated extensions of ancillary medical, especially nursing, roles. For instance, the Department of Health's (DoH 2006) declaration that, from May 2006, nurses may prescribe medicines – including some controlled drugs – questions what precisely the nursing role is. For notwithstanding the initial fanfare, nurse prescribing will still require close liaison with doctors, the nursing task being to adjust existing dosages to service user needs, the financial savings coming from the absent medic. Of course, psychiatric nurses have *always* influenced medical prescribing. However, reconfiguring this into a statutory right enshrines the shifting power bases of both professions. It also alters relationships with patients by removing the nurse as watchdog for their welfare. To whom will responsibility for patients' interests now fall if dosages are too high or when patients refuse drugs altogether? Pro-prescribers will respond that dosages are unlikely to be too high given nurses' increasing pharmaceutical knowledge. But it doesn't follow that enhanced knowledge of drugs promotes less prescribing; if anything, it suggests an even heavier faith in drugs and their positive effects.

THE MEDICAL DIMENSION

Actually, it was ever thus. When nurses picked up thermometers so did their medical progression begin, although the routinisation of their use – B/P & TPRs twice daily – established this as an *assistance* activity and nursing autonomy remained in check. For most nurses, this will remain the case. However, the reworking of some psychiatric nurses, via prescribing, and within contexts of diminished doctors' powers, is becoming a fact. The stethoscope (worn as a necklace) has become as iconic of nurses' persona as it is of doctors', a visible declaration of medical ascendancy if ever there was one. Psychiatric nurses lack the stethoscope, true, but the prescription pad is now theirs and an ancient medical prerogative is abridged in their favour.

Another facet of change is a diminishing status of professionals in managing affairs within organisations such as the NHS. In a post-Thatcher age, managerialism remains king, its self-perpetuation dependent on such fripperies as refocusing the patient role as 'consumer', introducing 'dignity nurses' and creating managerial subunits to facilitate these.

> *"Management used to be a process by which you kept the company doing whatever it was meant to be doing. Now it has become a product. Most companies ... exist to create, maintain and expand management. Management is their product. Management is what they do."*

(Bywater 2004, pp. 56–57)

With exponential rises in medical technology, hospitals have become even greater citadels of cure and this requires administration. Therefore, the rise of the 'medicrat' and his constantly breaking down computer, the ubiquity of targets, reductions in waiting times and, ultimately, redundant nurses when the misspending of the medicrats needs to be offset. In all of this, the nursing profession plays but a consultancy role, affairs being driven by forces beyond their control.

DEFINING NURSING

This is not easy. However, nurse education's entry into the university provides a starting point. Certainly, this move reflected assumptions that nursing was now a profession, not in the old sense of moral standing but, now, as one of the learned professions. Indeed, modern nursing staunchly rejects angelic imagery and even concepts of vocation become embarrassing. A corollary of this rejection is the frantic search for a knowledge base reflecting the 'new' profession and its postulates. Since medicine could not provide this, given its prior ownership by another group, something else was needed and what transpired was a mixture of 'person centredness' and 'holistic care'. Henceforth, nursing would be a 'caring profession' devoid of the crudities of pathology, drugs, syringes or ECT machines. Leaving aside the curious implication that nurses had hitherto *not* 'cared' there came a flood of academic papers (mostly rhetorical) pronouncing an epistemologically independent nursing. Not since the ancient Greeks has rhetoric dominated learned discourse, and nurses have been very good at it. Endemic to this rhetoric has been the anti-reasoning championed by French philosopher Michel Foucault (1971) but which is scorned by those who place a scientific discourse above all others. Trying to hold the tension between these two viewpoints has sometimes proved difficult, as readers will see.

A PREPARATORY WORD ABOUT FOUCAULT

In trying to explain Foucault in real terms, we need to understand that from about the mid-18th-century, medical perceptions begin to shift to the body as the focus of interest in the sense that man becomes the object as well as the subject of knowledge. Whereas before, medicine had configured the body as an empty space into which, on the basis of abstract classifications of morbidity, illnesses might be projected, 18th-century medicine made anatomical investigations feasible, the medical gaze now itemising *parts* of the body, visualising illness through pathological, clinical and post-mortem analysis. Equally has 19th-century psychiatry gazed upon the brain as the organising centre of persons; henceforth, madness would be defined less from its experience and more from an evolving science of brains. Thus did rationality cost the 'madman' his 'village idiot' status; now, 'the mad' would be segregated by a psychiatric discourse that declares them to be without reason.

THE FIVE SECTIONS

The ideas listed at the beginning of this introduction are deployed throughout five sections which illuminate concerns and applications particular to each but with elements of generalisation added on where appropriate. The summaries of these sections pinpoint their more salient features, explaining, justifying and preparing the reader for the wider discussions that follow.

SECTION 1:   A WORD ABOUT RESEARCH AND DIARIES

Two research paradigms, each differing radically about what counts as evidence, affect alternate influences on nursing research.

In general, I defend the appropriateness of both qualitative and quantitative methods – depending on the nature of the research question – while castigating qualitative researchers who espouse continental philosophy (see Ch. 3), asserting a position whereby everything is rendered equal.

> "*The Simpsons is an Anglo-Saxon comedic take on the existentialism which in France takes on a more tragic hue. The satirical cartoon world is essentially a philosophical one because to work, it needs to reflect accurately by abstracting it, distilling it, illuminating it more brightly than realist fiction can. It is no coincidence that the most philosophical cultural product of our time is a comic cartoon and why its creator, Matt Groening, is the true heir of Plato, Aristotle and Kant.*"

(Baggini 2006, p. 27)

The hint that this works better in France is happily taken. However, this is not everyone's view and that such buffoonery informs the reasoning of certain psychiatric nursing researchers is cause for concern. However, I have attempted to provide a balanced picture by means of critically overhauling elements from both approaches whilst, in addition, placing the research chapters against an exploratory background of what psychiatric nursing is. Little passes for viable practice now that is not evidence based, by which is meant researched in some or other form. However, too much has been assumed about the relevant powers of different research forms and too much taken for granted about what constitutes, for example, evidence itself. My emphasis on research therefore forms an appropriate opening to this book.

SECTION 2: CAN THERE BE A NURSING ETHICS?

These chapters address the ethics of organised psychiatric power and the roles of nurses. Fundamentally, can there *be* a nursing ethics that differs from its medical counterpart? I think not since distinct orientations would require arbitration and how to achieve *that* other than by who carries most occupational clout? Nevertheless, a nursing ethics is asserted by many, its essentials typically locked into concepts of caring. Chapter 7 casts doubt on this by questioning what it is that nurses care *about*. The chapters are grounded in practical events (see Ch. 5) largely because 'pure' ethics can be perceived as unworldly. In addition, I have opted for topics that are contemporary and important such as control and restraint, patients' rights, racism and institutional power.

SECTION 3:   ETHNICITY, RACE AND THE PADDIES

Issues of ethnicity challenge psychiatry's protestations of objectivity, its claims to abjure value judgements when treating patients. Further, as psychiatric service users become influential, assessing how they may *take* responsibility for their particular identities becomes important. Ethnicity is a touchy but increasingly relevant subject in mental health care (Fernando 2003, Littlewood & Lipsedge 1982). Although ethnicity overlaps with race the two are different, although precise definitions are elusive: both are contested terms. Recently, ethnic studies have usefully addressed issues of mental distress and recovery and in this section I have cohered my chapters around Irish people and especially their experiences as immigrants. This has the advantage of siphoning attention from black and Asian people as problem groups, thus diminishing the worrying propensity to see groups different from one's own as 'exotically salient' (Littlewood 1985) and thus sociologically significant. Irish people become an apt group, by which to examine overlaps of ethnicity and race within British contexts since they share a racial inheritance but differ along ethnic grounds. In addition, mental illness captures and expresses their history, conscious and imagined, as immigrants, living within cultures they only partly comprehend. Thus, such things as migrancy, poverty, poor health practices and their correlates with mental distress are examined. Importantly, the issues raised can be generalised to any ethnicity but particularly those seeking, as once the Irish did, the comforts of asylum.

Famine

For Irish people, no phase of history burns darker than the famines of the 1840s. By this is not meant some facile 'cultural memory syndrome' where ancient tragedies are seen as metaphors for psychological distress, but that such events become the part-fictional remembrances of people, affecting how they are ill, and especially when they live amongst those whom they blame for their problems. Remembrances are multi-faceted: there is the fact of many famine dead but, more so, how British governments responded to it. Such responses are frequently depicted as malevolent and in Chapter 9 you will discover the terms 'Irish holocaust', 'genocide' and the like. Although serious historians shrink from these terms, they often emerge in popular culture. The singer Sinead O'Connor (1994), for example, has a song called *Famine* with the words 'there *was* no famine', which is implicitly accusatory since, further on, she sings 'meat fish vegetables were shipped out of the country under armed guard'. A more accurate picture, these days, would run:

> *"In reality British government reactions to the famine were certainly not motivated by some genocidal impulse, but were at best insensitive, inefficient and ineffective."*

(Howe 2002, p. 38)

Observe, the only note of criticism above is 'insensitive', everything else being attributed to administrative failure. Personally, I am sceptical of 'holocaust' and 'genocide', their function probably servicing ideologically motivated ends. Yet 'scholarly accounts' of 'insensitivity' or 'inefficiency' do not mitigate the thousands who died. That these deaths pre-empted a 'Celtic melancholia' is, however, questionable. However, a case is made within these chapters for linking cultural identity to the experience of distress, social breakdown and even psychosis.

SECTION 4: EDUCATION, EDUCATION, EDUCATION

What is the role of contemporary nursing students; are they, in a Kantian sense, the means towards profiting educational elites? How do global markets and technology affect what students are taught and do they have any say in this? How is the role of women implicated in educational change in a still largely female occupation?

These questions underpin moves from the 'university of culture' to the 'virtual university' where knowledge is no longer owned by the scholarly few but is instead disseminated to the many by globalisation and its offspring technology. British universities sell education abroad, for instance, and rely significantly upon overseas students for financial income at home. Universities are now less reservoirs for definable cultures and more corporate entities generating and packaging courses aimed at customer and service/industrial groups. Naturally, tension exists between those wishing to retain the 'culture' university and those who see purchasers' requirements – for example NHS trusts – as important. For example, with the 'virtual university' (Robins & Webster 2002) pure knowledge is replaced with 'performative', where pure science gives way to scientific *outcomes* leading to patents, products and profits. In psychiatric nursing, dissimilarities exist between such performative knowledge as reliance on drugs rather than on understanding distress in subjective (potentially profit-losing) ways. Another product uptake by British psychiatric nurses has been American humanistic ideas and, more recently, more home-grown activities such as cognitive behaviour therapy.

But, mostly, my criticisms point at corporatist universities cramming their campuses with students, partly because governments want this but also for financial gain. For some universities, the nursing numbers are particularly remunerative but, at a deeper level, nurses symbolise value of knowledge for its own sake as against what transfers into work and economy. In fact, nursing students uniquely reflect how the 'university of culture' has led to the 'university of the masses' and Chapter 16 asks if more students lead to diminishing standards.

More means worse

The 'more means worse' debate has festered in higher education since first mooted in *Encounter* magazine, by the novelist Kingsley Amis, in July 1959. Although originally machines for generating church, civil service, medical and legal fodder, universities had more recently become centres of intellectual thought seemingly impervious to their outside worlds. Those favouring the latter are understandably appalled by university expansionism into professional and service fields. Yet, that universities were ever completely self-serving and devoted to purity of thought may be wishful thinking. At the same time, until about the 1970s, that's how they were perceived, entry into their hallowed groves assiduously pegged to top scorers in examinations or entrance tests – and with linkages to class and privilege.

By the 1990s, this had exploded into a carnival of activities with colleges embracing 'widening participation' schemes, polytechnics re-baptised as universities, courses dissected into manageable modules and burgeoning entry figures. There was concern about alleged 'dumbing down' of qualifications to facilitate entry for less able students. A politics of 'social inclusion' saw governments pander to electorates, identifying this, that or the other group as potential members of an escalating meritocracy. You too can be a university student or you too can prescribe psychiatric drugs and so forth. No need to fear examinations, failure at which might reduce self-esteem; we will arrange for you to have project-work and home-based assessments. And when you join the university we will treat you nicely, assume that your every complaint – you are, after all, our customers – is valid. The point of this is that by assuming that people are not up to scratch, the academic goalposts are then changed, so that the content of what is taught can sometimes become meaningless (Furedi 2004). Recently, when asked to 'teach' psychiatric nursing students, I discovered each of them had brought along a personal interest (for example, metal work); they then demonstrated this interest before asking the rest of us to have a go. It in no way differed from the primary school activity 'bring and show' although I believe that in educationalist circles it is called 'action learning sets'.

Yet, on reflection, why should including non-traditional subjects – tourism studies let's say – cause concern? And, if the wider population cannot acquire top school grades, what else *but* to make them more achievable? Also, why *should* examination grades be the only measure of university potential, especially in an era of relativism, pace Foucault, where everyone must have a place in the sun? Here, in a nutshell, lies the genesis of access courses, NVQ Gateways and assessment standards of questionable rigour. So does more *really* mean worse or, as John Radford (1997) suggests, does it simply mean 'different'? Read on and find out.

SECTION 5:   DRUGS, EUPHEMISMS AND CYBORGS

This section's chapters are metaphors for what may happen as psychiatric nursing proceeds. My threefold purpose is to ask if the claims of bio-pharmacologists should be taken at face value or if we should prize 'person centredness' however derivatively vague it sometimes seems. Second, why do some people misuse language, inducing us to believe what they want us to, even when we do not wish to? Third, can we trust machines which claim to 'see' mental illness inside human brains? The metaphorical nature of these chapters suggests an other-worldliness but where speculation is becoming more and more feasible, especially, it is claimed, in fields such as schizophrenic brain imaging.

Drugs

Both legally and illegally we are a drugs culture. Drugs affect human thought, feeling and behaviour; they are also contentious in terms of their effectiveness. The story of how psychotropic drugs came to be overvalued is told here within the context of changes in nurse education and especially (see Ch. 18) how 'persuader language' came to bolster their 'magic bullet' status. That status influenced beliefs about the underlying biology of mental illness which reciprocally fed back into an expanding bio-techno-pharmacology. In fact, the power of the pharmaceutical role rests on a limited number of useful drugs, their success, in turn, resting on exaggerated claims of their usefulness. Another point is that psychotropic drugs *construct* many of the images of 'the schizophrenic': the facial grimacing, endless pacing up and down, muscular contractions and mouth dribbling. These drug-induced effects are what give us this picture, not illness itself.

Words, words, words

Language may be abused as part of the acquisition of power. Foucault (1971) suggests that language *is* power and we will examine what this means. Neither must we be misled by its shared usage when this occurs; sharing our jargon, for example with service users, may be merely to win their assent and cooperation. Chapter 19 deals with how we use words in a context of 'challenging behaviour' and what this term means. The fastidiousness of the DSM-IV is likewise criticised as the main culprit in systems thinking but there is also examined the 'false consciousness' associated with the largely uncritical uptake of American humanistic thinking, especially that of Carl Rogers (2003) and Patricia Benner (2001).

The cyborg

Machines are everywhere and don't we just love them. Apparently, some academics are about to publish a code of ethics for machines because, it seems, they are becoming too sophisticated (Habershon & Woods 2006). In an age when robots can plausibly be considered as crowd control operators or as helpers for the infirm elderly, this hardly surprises. Chapter 20 explores how this extends into psychiatry and how technology points towards ways of managing it.

Since the inception of philosopher Alan Turing's 'machine' (Ch. 20), human function has been studied analogous to computers and important theoretical questions have emerged. Allowing that computers can absorb new information suggests that if they utilised this information reflexively they could generate new material not initially programmed into them. Could the computer then be said to have a mind of its own?

My chapter on virtual systems discusses philosophical issues that most psychiatric nursing texts avoid. It explores technology designed to amplify biological systems and links this to questions about reality, knowledge and power. It asks if machines can 'think' and, if so, could they ever become psychotic? This may appear silly at first but when set within the 'mind–brain problem', and attempts at solving this through computer simulation, it acquires meaning. The point is that questions about schizophrenia are meaningless when isolated from how humans think generally and computers have been used extensively to look at the latter. For example, positivists have used technology to make it seem as if consciousness is a side issue. So that when schizophrenia is 'seen' in PET scan pictures, intrinsic consciousness becomes threatened as part of a general reductionism. As Glen Ward (2003, p.75) suggests:

> "The logical order of things might be that reality expresses itself through representations, but this has been turned upside down."

Depth has been succeeded by surface, and visual imagery is now a source of persuasion and control. It used to be that, following Goffman (1960), we struggled for identity through our occupations or through parenting or being Irish, American and so on. Today, we sit transfixed as our television screens portray searches for identity under the surgeon's knife or via looks or lifestyles considered OK by fashion gurus or proselytisers of the 'body beautiful' or whatever.

A word about *The Matrix* film which I introduce in Chapter 20. This film raises questions about identity and the notion of a post-human condition. Such a 'condition' is not to be taken literally, perhaps, but it does conjure a future that is intriguing at best and, at worst, perverse and threatening. We are already some way towards versions of the cyborg (or cybernetic organism), half man, half machine, where mind and body are redefined (Ward 2003) as more powerful than the 'merely' human. Think of pacemakers, mechanical hearts, body prosthetics, silicon implants, cosmetic surgery, dialysis machines, genetic engineering, plastic joints, contact lenses, surgically reconnected limbs, replacement faces. We may be years away from implanting brain parts but even without reaching that we still face questions of identity that are formidable enough.

References

Baggini J 2006 Pseud's corner. Private Eye 1160:27

Benner P 2001 From novice to expert. Dutton, New Jersey

Bywater M 2004 Lost worlds. Granta, London

Department of Health 2006 Independent nurse prescribing. Online. Available: http://www.dh.gov.uk/policyandguidance

Fernando S 2003 Cultural diversity, mental health and psychiatry. Brunner-Routledge, Hove

Foucault M 1971 Madness and civilization: a history of insanity in an age of reason. Tavistock, London

Furedi F 2004 Where have all the intellectuals gone? Continuum, London

Goffman E 1960 Asylums. Penguin, Harmondsworth

Habershon E, Woods R 2006 No sex please, robot, just clean the floor. The Sunday Times, June 18th, p. 11

Howe S 2002 Ireland and Empire. Oxford University Press, Oxford

Littlewood R 1985 An indigenous conceptualization of reactive depression in Trinidad. Psychiatric Medicine 15(2):275–281

Littlewood R, Lipsedge M 1982 Aliens and alienists. Penguin, Harmondsworth

O'Connor S 1994 Universal mother. Ensign/Chrysalis Music, London

Radford J 1997 The changing purposes of higher education. In: Radford J, Raaheim K, de Vries P et al (eds) Quantity and quality in higher education. Jessica Kingsley, London, pp. 7–47

Robins K, Webster F 2002 The virtual university? Oxford University Press, Oxford

Rogers C 2003 Client centred therapy. Constable, London

Ward G 2003 Teach yourself postmodernism. Hodder, London

A word about research and diaries

SECTION CONTENTS

1

Research: vocation, profession: which?

And always keep a hold of nurse
For fear of finding something worse

(Hilaire Belloc 1870–1953)

Before asking about the relevance of research to nursing, a more propitious question might be: 'what is nursing?' The word *nursing* covers a multitude of implications both overt and covert. Some believe that nurses have lost their way. *Sunday Times* columnist Melanie Phillips (1999), for instance, constantly reiterates the virtues of 'basic nursing' and wonders when nurses will eventually see sense and 'go back'. Go back to *what* is rarely made explicit but, generally, what is implied is the re-uptake of a housekeeping function, re-imposing task-oriented nursing full of order and hygiene. Critics, like Phillips, see the move of nurse education from hospital-based training schools into the universities as retrogressive, distracting nurses from a pre-ordained vocation to provide basic care and sustenance. The university move symbolises the chasm between nursing as a knowledge-based, even intellectual, activity or as a giving of 'basic nursing care' that reflected the *character* of nurses, their altruism, their dedication. Nothing wrong with that, perhaps, although redefining nursing as 'hands on' work requiring minimal theory and a didactic training based on received ideas is also problematic. It may be recalled that it was because of 'received learning' that the Robbins Committee (1963) firmly rejected nursing for inclusion within higher education frameworks. Nurse education remained disconnected to everything else, its certificates and diplomas, for example, utterly untransferable to other institutions or courses. It was precisely this educational abyss that provoked nurse educationalists to push for entry into higher education. What research there is, for this process, reflects division with those advocating academia tending to occupy prestigious institutions such as the Royal College of Nursing or the Department of Health, and with 'shop floor' opinions either unknown or else 'translated' by educationalists as probably favourable. Humphreys (1996) links the aspirations of nurse elitists to NHS reform generally with its myriad, changing, demands. More specifically, Mackay (1998), in a study of vocation and professionalism, found that many of her subjects favoured nursing qualities such as 'character' and not 'academia' and, although only a small number used the word 'vocation', the activities they perceived as nursing matched this concept. In addition, Mackay also noted how the professionalisers in nursing were few, mainly made up of educationalists and even smaller numbers of service leaders.

Be that as it may, educational changes seriously invigorated the scholarly instincts of many and considerable numbers of psychiatric nurses began to engage in research such that, whatever one's views about what nursing *ought* to be, there was no getting past the growing qualitative research activity of current British nurses. The qualitative emphasis is far from everybody's taste:

> *"There is something of an anti trial culture in nursing in the UK, where nurses seem particularly keen to adopt research designs which are clearly different from their medical colleagues. Thus, papers which argue for qualitative research in preference to [randomised controlled trials] RCTs abound."*

(Cullum 1997, p. 5)

Within the qualitative camp, the impression conveyed is of nursing as an educated (and educating) activity which questions and even seeks to undermine traditional practice. Now, everybody needs education and nurses are no different in wanting to test their practice against theories and ideas. However, it is remarkable how many first-level students protest that their courses are failing to provide what they see as the skills needed for 'basic nursing care'. Of course, what counts as 'basic nursing care' is elusive and it perplexes me that *students* know what it is, that they seem able to locate it within traditional practice rather than with theory or ideas. Observe how their beliefs about basic nursing solidify following exposure to practice, the latter reinforcing what, in practical settings, actually 'works'. What happens, I think, is that they come to the university vaguely aware that something is amiss, where requirements to engage academically feel intuitively odd. In a sense, they join the university but are not *of* it. Any subsequent intensification of philosophical and psychological theorising furthers the suspicion that something really *is* amiss and it is then that they start to exclaim: 'But I came here to be a nurse!' However, it is their clinical placements which confirm their initial instinct that classroom-based sociology is not what matters. And, anyway, the classroom is a lame duck experience: practice arenas, ultimately, are where promotion (or sanction) lies. Educationalists, of course, insist that pre-registration education equips students more complexly than before, that it provides them with *analytical* skills. However, for many students, theories embalmed in classroom curricula are a rite of passage which simply have to be endured prior to everyday practice.

THE PROBLEM

This is skating on thin ice but I do not think that nursing, given its nature, can be researched. This is not to devalue what nurses do but to reiterate that no necessary relationship exists between explanation and appreciation. Lacking explanation, one can still advance nursing as an intuitively good, praiseworthy, even noble, profession. However, this is hardly what nurse scholars do. Quite the contrary; discomfited by the nobility tag which insinuates vocation, they have instead set out to define nursing as knowledge based, its skills and practice conducive to empirical investigation. However, they have done this from positions which smack more of wishful thinking than any agreed formulation of definition of what nursing is.

For if there exists a basic nursing care, then either the 'nursing' or the 'care' must be dropped because they constitute a tautology. We are then left with basic nursing but I think that we can also drop the 'basic' because unless we can define the 'nursing', trying to define basic nursing is putting the cart before the horse. Attempting to research what cannot be defined is puzzling, to put it mildly, and it looks as if nurse researchers have been engaged in underhand practices in trying to do so. The current preoccupation of some academics with RCTs, for instance, quickly exposes some core problems when applying these to nursing problems. Ideally, RCTs are most useful with data that can be manipulated as independent and dependent variables, for example in agricultural research, where they originated. With people, they ideally suit problems that involve bio-physical-chemical equations; double-blind drug trials, for instance, where criteria for success or failure are pre-specified and measured both independently and objectively. It would hardly do, for instance, to experimentally administer psychotropic medication to subjects and then inquire some time later how they were feeling. They might be feeling better so as to please you or feeling worse so as to keep your attention. No: something more inhuman seems called for, some way of randomly measuring things which deletes the subjective views of those most involved.

This contradicts those who either claim to use RCTs in nursing or who argue that this is what that nurse researchers ought to do. The contradiction stems from the incompatibility of a process which is essentially about context stripping and minimising individual differences as against a historical nursing that prizes these qualities to a greater or lesser extent. Watching RCT nurses as they try to wriggle their way out of this dilemma becomes an education in itself.

NURSES AND RCTS

When nurse researchers do RCTs they typically substitute for 'nursing care' some other type of intervention. For example, they might randomly establish groups of people where Group 1 receives one treatment, Group 2 gets another while a third group gets no treatment at all, thus fulfilling some of the methodological requirements of the RCT. There are, however, huge problems – typically glossed over – when setting up these 'random' groups, not least of which is the issue of consent. If, for example, one group consists of people with psychotic disorders then how does consent to treatment work, particularly in experimental contexts in which some of the subjects receive no treatment at all? RCT aficionados, unsurprisingly, deal with this problem by randomising treatments amongst non-randomly selected groups. The question of randomly allocating *subjects* within these groups or the difficulties in determining their representativeness – given that subjects will often be ill in ways that are themselves ill-defined – are also neglected issues. However, notwithstanding the technical difficulties, the issue is that we are talking here about *treatments,* not nursing. For example, in a mental health RCT, the study might involve a comparison between drug therapy as against cognitive behaviour therapy or no therapy at all. The *nursing* dimension is conveniently side-stepped and understandably so, for if nursing is to do with relationships then this puts the qualitative cat squarely among the quantitative pigeons. Nursing, to my mind, unless operationalised as a discrete therapy, is just not researchable under randomised conditions. Part of the reason why these studies have gone ahead – even, sometimes, trumpeted as the spearhead of a scientific nursing – is that many nurses see little or no contradiction between the nurse as therapist, whether the therapy in question is prescribing drugs or implementing behaviourism, or the nurse as basic practitioner. This might be a sustainable position where the therapy is but one of a number of activities performed by a nurse.

However, where it becomes the mainstay of the nurses' role, it becomes difficult to continue to assert its identity as nursing.

THE QUALITATIVE DOMAIN

The essential point of difference between quantitative and qualitative research is that the latter allows for an examination of relationships; even verbal data that contradict the research hypothesis, if there is one, need not be a problem. With this type of research you can evaluate relationships to your heart's content except that you are then faced with persuading your audience that your work is scientific. Having used both approaches, there are some things to be said both for and against each of them. First, the deficiencies of qualitative studies are very real when asserted to be scientific; their advantage is that they can open up the internal meanings people attach to things, the manner by which they make sense of – and act within – their social worlds. Quantitative research, alternatively, despite its dependency on empiricism, is best at deciphering questions about the physical world: it is materialist in its execution and its design. As such, it is woefully unable to map attitudinal, belief or emotional behaviours. Hence its redundancy in respect of nursing when conceptualised as interpersonal, ethical or even spiritual. There is no third way, by the way. Attempts to merge irreconcilable approaches to research are both misguided and confusing. For example, grafting numerical data onto human narratives adds nothing; conversely, obtaining personal views about life experiences adds little to our knowledge of the physical world. It may of course be possible to define problems operationally both in physical and psychological terms – people's experiences of heart arrhythmias, for instance, where different kinds of data combine well and can be useful. However, research questions ought to invite such two-pronged approaches and should not be embarked upon so as to augment the scholarly respectability of one or other method.

Lastly, it is not surprising that debate on these questions moved from the psychology profession in the 1950s and 1960s to psychiatric nursing in the 1980s, the opposing qualitative and quantitative camps becoming virulent at times. The virulence is not just about differences between methods but – like the British debate on 'keeping the pound' – goes much deeper: it is about the nature of the profession itself. Is nursing a *basic* profession? This poses problems: base things rarely amount to much and nurses run considerable risks whenever they call for a 'back to basics' approach. Undoubtedly, some nurses regard their work as 'common sense' and can become intolerant or indifferent to what they see as professional posturing or grandstanding. Even less do they cherish esoteric philosophies, preferring instead more pragmatic responses to practicalities. This begs the question of whether nursing is a 'proper' profession at all: that is, does it compare with disciplines such as medicine and law? Or is it too practice based, too preoccupied with the day-to-day exigencies of serving patients' fundamental needs? But even if this is conceded, many nurses are still involved in decision making, engaging with patients in ways that require reflection and analysis.

Perhaps nursing can encompass both dimensions. After all, the base activities of legal soliciting (messy divorces/house conveyancing) go comfortably hand-in-hand with the be-wigged barrister-led activities at the bar of the Old Bailey. Indeed, most professions have little problem subsuming disparate activities under their (wider) professional mantle. Nursing, however, has never easily encompassed differentially trained and/or paid practitioners, different portals of entry. In the case of enrolled nurses (ENs), for instance, these constituted a challenge to the claims of 'new nursing' to academic and professional status. In response, ENs were quickly 'converted' to registered status even though, before, they had competently performed the staff nurses' function when required. Notwithstanding these difficulties, it may be that some reconfiguration of the past is needed to free us from ambivalence and disarray. For example, why not have basic nursing performed by baseline nurses and leave the 'higher profession' bits to those with academic qualifications? If the latter agreed to call themselves by some other title, this might also help. Some, having adopted various therapeutic roles, are doing this already. Given that professionalism is about ascendancy and ownership, naturally those who aspire to greater professional standing will seek to redefine themselves. But trying to define what *nursing* is, as distinct from assuming new roles, will not help us establish a viable identity. This is because the essence of nursing is indefinable and such studies which do lay claim to its definition, as I have shown, are based on subtle redefinitions of function. Research programmes by nurses are simply studies by people who continue to award themselves the title nurse: it is hardly nursing research if there is no such thing as nursing. In fairness, this is a contested view.

LOCUS OF UNITY

In 1998, Philip Ross denied my contention that psychiatric nursing lacked a 'locus of unity' and that what he called 'the restoration and/or enhancement of rational autonomy' (to patients) constituted 'a single qualitative end' (Ross 1998, p. 183) by which nursing could be defined. He placed his response in a context of forced psychiatric treatments so as to suggest that nurses, acting as patients' 'advocates', fulfil a uniquely nursing role. However, there are problems with this: typically, in Britain, nurses are employed by the state and to a much lesser extent by private providers. In either case, though, they acquire occupational responsibility and, while this does not obligate them towards slavish or unethical behaviour, they are bound to the collective organisational codes of their respective institutions; their room for advocacy is going to be limited. Also, from what we know of nursing history, to postulate advocacy as a central concern of nurses seems ambitious. Who, for instance, could deny that nurses have, over the years, helped sustain medical conceptions of psychiatric disorder and its treatment, that they have played Sancho Panza to the medical quest?

Naming things is the first prerequisite of research and for most purposes, regardless of what quantifiers say, everyday language will suffice. But nurses still face a sticky wicket inasmuch as it becomes difficult to nail down exactly what is to be researched. Impaled upon the evidence-based demand that they account for their service, nurses may have little choice but to research its basic assumptions, the uniqueness of its input to care. But it is hamstrung in this by its curricular failure to declare an essentialist position which could be researched. An issue of exclusivity may highlight this: the Royal College of Nursing has for years discussed the question of whether to admit nursing auxiliaries to its membership, with many in favour, many against (they did so in 2000 provided the applicant had basic vocational qualifications). Those in favour, I suspect, saw little difference between the work of auxiliaries and what ought to be the work of those properly qualified. In my view, this is a perfectly defensible perspective albeit an expression of forlorn hope given the reality of staff nurses as 'mini doctors'. Now turn your mind to the Royal College of Physicians or even Psychiatrists: can anyone imagine the non-qualified being accepted for membership of these? Those who see the contradiction here will (a) seek to rid nursing of the enrolled nurse status and (b) oppose any entry of auxiliaries to the Royal College of Nursing. Nursing research then must needs navigate its way through and within these ambiguities and precarious positions. So far it has done this by advancing claims to professional inclusion, so as to deal with its perceived traditions of handmaiden and playing second fiddle to medics. But tub thumping about professional status and 'new' nursing knowledge is not enough: indeed, it becomes embarrassing the more you think about how these are used to circuitously amplify each other while ignoring the internal inconsistencies of each.

References

Cullum N 1997 Identification and analysis of randomised control trials in nursing: a preliminary study. Quality in Health Care 6(1):2–6

Humphreys J 1996 English nurse education and the reform of the National Health Service. Journal of Education Policy 11(6):655–659

Mackay L 1998 Nursing: will the idea of vocation survive? In: Abbott P, Meerabeau L (eds) The sociology of the caring professions. UCL Press, London, pp. 54–72

Phillips M 1999 How the college girls destroyed nursing. The Sunday Times, January 10th, p. 13

Robbins Committee on Higher Education 1963 Cmnd 2154. HMSO, London

Ross P 1998 The self and compulsory treatment. In: Edwards S D (ed) Philosophical issues in nursing. Macmillan Press, Basingstoke, pp. 183–199

2

Critiquing the gold standard in research: a personal view

All that glisters is not gold

(William Shakespeare, *Merchant of Venice*, II, vii)

The term 'evidence-based practice' (EBP) has become a cornerstone of contemporary health care. Enshrined in the workings of organisations such as the National Institute for Health and Clinical Excellence (NICE 2006) its influence is felt across a wide array of medical practice including psychiatric care. The term also carries great rhetorical force, a downside of which has been a lack of inquiry about what the term implies, of what actually counts as evidence. A commonly used definition is provided by Sackett et al (1996, p. 71):

> *"The conscientious, explicit and judicious use of current best evidence in making decisions about the care of individuals."*

While having the advantage of succinctness, it still leaves open the question of what evidence is. The perceived necessity for EBP reflected concerns about medical and surgical provision and the conviction that practice based on clinical judgement could be underpinned by standardised or factually based data.

Fairly quickly, EBP came to be viewed as conceptually linked to empirical, specifically quantitative factors, and with qualitative work seen as somehow second rate, anecdotal and 'soft'. Clearly, such a narrow empiricism would limit the range of much psychiatric nursing research which requires its evidence base to include an experiential dimension.

KINDS OF QUESTIONS

What counts as evidence depends on the questions to which answers are sought, the contexts in which questions occur and the purpose or ends to which they are put. For example, in judicial settings the subjectivity of witnesses challenges the court's quest for precision and nowhere is this more obvious than when juries confront the biased summaries of duelling lawyers and not always impartial judges. The process can hardly be called scientific; even the rigour of judicial rules governing evidence hardly counteracts the preconceived notions of your average jury member. It is a sobering thought that if a jury was substituted or even partly substituted with other jurors, alternative verdicts might well ensue. It is of course possible that the more tangible the evidence, the less this will happen; nevertheless, judicial procedures are imperfect as none-too-rare instances of miscarried justice show.

Similar problems beset qualitative researchers: just like jurors, so too are research audiences asked to accept subjective interpretations acquired through observations and interviews. Do such interpretations pass the 'good evidence' test? For instance, why should subjects in qualitative studies be believed? Might they not be lying so as to impress or conceal? Concepts of 'social desirability' are well established in the psychological literature (Fisher 1993) and, for many, political correctness has a strong purchase on how people behave. Being a subject in qualitative research does not confer immunity from self-deception, confusion or even mendacity. Also, as LaPierre (1934) convincingly showed, attitudes do not necessarily correspond with actions or vice versa so that assertions, by subjects, that they would or would not believe or act in certain ways may not constitute serious evidence.

FAIR CRITICISMS

I believe that such criticisms carry weight because the development of qualitative theory has isolated itself from broader traditions of sociological and psychological research. Nevertheless, subjective investigations are necessary in psychiatric research; indeed, given the experiential dimension of psychological problems, they may be the only way of yielding results that make sense of nursing as an interpersonal enterprise. This distances nursing from bio-techno-quantitative constructs, placing it instead within the humanities where its necessary dependence on everyday language fits. Whether or not this is a problem depends upon your point of view. One of the reasons that NICE (2006) pushes cognitive behaviour therapy is not simply because it generates evidence-based outcomes but, as well, for its capacity to describe these statistically or in bullet point form. Whereas, even the most robust qualitative studies can only provide descriptive/narrative accounts which are rarely explanatory. Indeed, their qualitative reliance on the Queen's English alienates the scientifically minded amongst us. Theirs, however, is a naïve reading of what language can do. Discussing the use of everyday terms as explanatory mechanisms, philosopher Mary Midgley (2001, p. 11) states:

> "Words such as care, heart, spirit, sense, *[her emphasis]* are tools designed for particular kinds of work in the give-and-take of social life ... They are not a cheap substitute, an inadequate folk psychology, due to be replaced by the proper terms of the learned."

Further, in respect of some research questions – how pain is experienced, for example – I submit that scientific descriptors might be counterproductive, might detract from an area where personal testimony is paramount. For example, can the yardstick for pain assessment be anything other than the patient's own assessment, where, if he/she says that it hurts 'that much', then that is exactly how much it hurts?

In his short paper 'The nonsense of effectiveness' the late Don Bannister (1998) asserted that in much of what passes for psychotherapy the 'medical model' still rules. By this he meant that many still seek yardsticks or models for how people *should* behave or recover and so on. Responding to the charge that talking therapies were inefficient, he suggested that if we substituted any common term for 'psychotherapy', such as 'conversation', then (p. 218):

> "if you were asked how effective is conversation you would surely begin by questioning the question. As it stands it is nonsense."

He has a point. Even so, we are continuously challenged to produce evidence that conversations with patients are effective, as if some abstract schemata could account for what is or is not conversationally effective. The assumption seems to be that all communication be grounded in categorical terms. But what is neatly sidestepped is the place of silence in communication, the significance of touch or the less obvious non-verbal forms of contact. The issue is not about segregating scientific inquiry but to stress that what helps people deal with psychological distress evolves within the relationships that psychotherapies provide. These factors are difficult to elicit and it becomes difficult to link outcomes with precise antecedents in therapy. This is especially true where problems possess low visibility, for example problems that stem from existential dread or anomie where it becomes difficult to ascertain what has or has not been effective other than to share with one's client quiet assurances that change *has* occurred.

Advocates of evidence-based approaches, of course, are suspicious of this and make heavy weather of proving effectiveness. To return to Bannister (1998, p. 219):

> *"Are you really prepared to contend that your relationships, your love affairs, your enmities, your long standing dialogue with your uncle Albert – whether the effect be good, bad or chaotic – have been, in some strange sense, ineffective?"*

Admittedly, personal relationships do not constitute psychotherapy. If one seeks to help people with psychological difficulties there occurs *some* obligation to acknowledge that one *can* alleviate the problems, not perhaps in providing predictive outcomes but at least in the moral sense of believing that what one offers is helpful. That said, many therapists engage with patients in ways that do resemble loving relationships, seeking to harness the trust, mutual respect and acceptance that cultures such relationships.

COST

Demonstrating the effectiveness of helping – especially when cost is an issue – constitutes a moral imperative that needs to be balanced against other considerations. The financial cost of research can be used to blackmail nurse researchers away from qualitative work. This is especially the case for NHS nurses whose monies come from the public purse. However, differences in orientation will also reflect the kinds of psychological problems that are responded to. Contemporary fascination with cost-effective, evidence-based treatments acquires credence through in-built assumptions that particular problems merit more attention than others. Evidence-based practice seems best suited to disorders; such as schizophrenia or obsessive compulsive disorder; it appears less suited to disorganised or fragmented distress rooted in problems in living, to self-perceived low esteem or, even, difficulties in *being*. In fact, with hospital closures it became the case that many community psychiatric nurses (CPNs) had built up case loads of just such 'problems in living' patients. By the 1990s concerns were being expressed that such work was being undertaken at the expense of psychotic patients. These concerns formed the basis for an influential study (Gournay & Brooking 1994) which tested the efficacy of CPNs across different categories of clients. The study reported, somewhat negatively, that CPNs should refocus their energies towards psychotic patients and away from those deemed 'less ill'. In particular, the CPNs' penchant for those called 'the worried well' was challenged.

Further, nurse educationalists were encouraged to recognise the importance of interventions of 'proven effectiveness' and transmit these to students. An important implication of this work was that CPNs might better occupy their time – given the state of NHS funding – working with those fitting the descriptor 'serious and enduring' mental illness. That NHS administrators were beginning to accept the reality of rationing made it opportune to question what CPNs were doing, who were their target groups.

The issue is not about denying the importance of categorising psychological problems, but that abstract yardsticks of distress are questionable. True, an adolescent may take up considerable psychotherapeutic time when he is 'merely' having difficulties with girls. The reality, these days, is that he is probably affluent since psychotherapy is now predominantly a private-sector activity. And, even if he is poor, arguably the CPNs' emphasis should still be on psychotic and organically impaired patients, not helping young men with 'difficulties'. CPNs are, after all, *nurses*, a title that carries implications of tending the *sick* and, inversely, is the young man with relationship problems sick? Perhaps not, but supposing he is permitted to drift away from therapy, suppose his low esteem turns to self-loathing, a loathing that leads him to the brink of self-harm? Durkheim's classic text *Suicide* (1989) is premised on exactly such a concept of 'anomie', the individual cut adrift from his/her fellows, even when in the midst of urban sprawl and congestion. So that if economics drive CPNs towards certain categories of patients shouldn't they acknowledge this and spare us the specious reasoning that priorities are prioritised because some are less worthy than others.

INSTITUTIONALISM

Surely Bannister was right to argue that only by valuing the personal can we hope to confront institutional forms of care. By institutional psychiatry is meant not just in-patient systems but the corrosive attitudes and practices that characterise psychiatric provision generally (Martin 1984, Stanley & Penhale 1999). Adhering too closely to received ideas about what constitutes evidence and avoiding questions about its nature deprives patients of the benefits that accrue from such questions. Suppose, for example, 'the evidence' suggests that a particular psychoactive drug is effective. Does it follow that administering it to people is without ethical issue? Where it is refused, does it follow that this refusal be denied the status of evidence? Institutional psychiatry, however, dismisses such refusals as constituting the clinical phenomenon 'non-compliance' (Lowry 1998).

That drug refusals represent pleas for survival or even expressions of self-concern receives short shrift. Equally, those who argue that non-compliance is merely a label and not a denial of the reasoning behind the refusal are mistaken since labelling cuts across individuality to begin with, denying the evidence of the senses, of what patients say, what they assert and do. Indeed, the essence of denial lies not in ignoring the patients' claims but in turning them into signs and symptoms.

HELPING PERSONS

Bannister (1998, p. 219, his emphasis) went on to say that:

> *"if our experience of psychological therapy makes sense to us, that is to say we can see reasons why we have been of no help to this person or some help to that person and we find that we can develop our understanding through our work, we are likely to continue to work this way* whatever the literature may say.*"*

His last paragraph reads (p. 220):

> *"My contention is that we should work as psychologists not as psychic paramedics. Our language, research methods and theory should be drawn from psychology and not from an imprisoning imitation of medical treatment studies."*

If true for psychologists, how doubly true it is for psychiatric nurses! Before moving on, I would labour the point that it is not that therapists do not form relationships with their patients. It is that one ought not denigrate those who do this *for its own sake*. To belittle work that falls outside of empirical evidence is mistaken. Actually, there are occasions when qualitative research exposes the deficiencies of quantitative work. Jolley et al (1998), for example, used a RCT approach to examine nursing interventions designed to rehabilitate heart attack victims. When the study yielded statistically insignificant results, Wiles (1998) qualitatively interviewed 25 of the Jolley et al subjects, identifying factors of acquisition and loss of trust deemed to be of clinical significance.

KEEPING UP WITH THE JONESES

On the principle of 'if you can't beat them, join them, some practitioners and researchers have embarked on mixed research designs. The process is called triangulation and, while interesting in part, can lead to emulating scientific research for appearances' sake. This occurs due to beliefs that verbally grounded research is somehow inferior to the numerical standing of the other. However, qualitative, approaches are less a research method and more a world perspective which entails, in part, a challenge to the dominance of physical science. Yet, curiously, qualitative findings are often presented so as to resemble scientific work. Thus, instead of validity and reliability we get 'creditability' and 'auditability' and so on. Even psychiatric work that centralises patients' experiences is still minded to present outcomes in an 'evidence-based results' style. In Loewenthal's (1999) view, such preoccupations reflect continuing fascination with objective thought and the impressiveness of science. This amplifies the respect which our culture accords to intellect over emotion whose expression – other than within acceptably defined limits – is usually suspect. The parents who visit their child's school for mid-term report are likely to be impressed when told that Jimmy is a pleasant lad who applies himself with great effort to the task at hand. Their pleasure will increase when informed that he shows artistic merit, that his paintings are charming, that he plays the violin quite well. But watch Mum and Dad's eyes gleam when told that Jimmy is heading for straight A grades and may be 'university material'. The fact is, in our society, we place a high premium on intelligence and the acquisition of knowledge and skills. Notwithstanding this, educationalists, at all levels, have favoured experiential approaches – an ideology of education that is only now changing – and nurse education has also long followed this route. However, concepts of skills and outcome measures have now been re-imposed at national level and the pressure is on to change yet again.

Qualitative research or 'people evidence' contradicts in principle such abstract skills frameworks. Loewenthal (1999) quotes Kierkegaard (1941, p. 67):

> *"Whilst objective thought is indifferent to the thinking subject and his existence, the subjective thinker is an existing individual essentially interested in his own thinking, existing as he does in thought. His thinking has therefore a different type of reflection, namely the reflection of inwardness, of possession, by virtue of which it belongs to the thinking subject and no one else."*

However, psychiatric nurses are too large and heterogeneous a group to settle for one type of explanation; some will favour a scientific view or they will insist that their qualitative perspective *is* scientific. This is mistaken. Whilst the quest for empirical 'evidence' is necessary when testing physical treatments, nurses can hardly eschew the lived testimony of patients. Even where patients lack the capacity for objective thought, this by no means renders their statements unworthy as evidence. The formation of the Hearing Voices Network (Coleman & Smith 1997) testifies to the refusal of psychiatric professionals to take seriously the subjective status of psychiatric patients. Nurses have played their part in such refusals largely by their preparedness to act as intermediaries for them. However, increasingly, psychiatric nurses are taking service users seriously, welcoming them as participants in service and educational activities. Whether their participation will favour more comprehensive concepts of what counts as evidence remains to be seen. Will a measure of scepticism about what is meant by evidence emerge so as to allow for varieties of clinical practice rather than locking everything up within cognitive behavioural domains?

A FINAL SWIPE

RCTs are powerless to assess relationship formation and change. Rather do they construe therapeutic relationships as uncontrollable variables to be minimised or evicted from consideration altogether. Instead, RCTs investigate the difference between discrete interventions: between, for instance, a drug, a cognitive behavioural intervention and no intervention at all. In effect, as psychiatrist Matthew Hotopf (2002, p. 328) notes:

> *"The majority of RCTs in psychiatry have been designed to answer a relatively narrow set of questions predominantly related to psychopharmacological treatments. There have been very few RCTs to assess more complex aspects of health care which may be no less important than the drugs we prescribe. Examining ... professional relationships and boundaries are what non RCT research is about."*

The qualitative research alternative explores the nature of relationships: one thinks of empathic understanding in Rogerianism or transference in psychoanalysis. True, these are difficult to research and the current advice from NICE is to give both of them a wide berth. However, while it's true that psychoanalysis is not effective with, let's say, compulsive obsessive disorder (Malan 1995) and cognitive behaviour therapy is, to continue to rule out non-cognitive approaches generally is short sighted. Different problems need to be looked at in different ways; no one possesses 'the gold standard', that vulgar emblem of one-upmanship. Qualitative approaches have their own purchase on human affairs, for example the contention of feminist critiques that psychiatric treatments actually denigrate the political and social status of women. Of course RCT advocates respond that, by definition, RCTs fall outside subjective notions of what it is to be human (or female!), that they are not about the business of assessing experience. True. However, psychiatric nurses disfavour themselves when, collating such experience, they then convert to an evidence structure that emulates experimental designs. There is much in the world that, given a chance, will account for itself in recognisable terms. Some of life's most important stuff doesn't need evidence. Having introduced logical positivism to British audiences – the belief that every word must have a recognisable referent to the physical world or else be disowned as useless metaphysics – Sir Frederick Ayer (1936) was subsequently asked how he would respond if his wife told him she loved him: what *evidence* would he require in support of her assertion? For once, the great philosopher was lost for words. Indeed, one wonders how cognitivists generally would deal with this 'problem'. What proof would they seek, what corroborative (collaborative?) evidence would they demand to support the notion of love? This gap between the tangible and that which is merely apprehended leads to a loss of patience among those who insist that the non-tangible is important. For:

> *"Lovers and madmen have such seething brains, such shaping fantasies, that apprehend, more than cool reason ever comprehends."*

> (Shakespeare 1948, Act 5, Sc. 1)

Anthony Burgess adds significantly to an understanding of how this works. Reflecting on Defoe's *A Journal of the Plague Year* (1978) he comments:

> *"The journal is unique in that, accepting it as fiction, every generation has also taken it as history. Despite the intrusions of hearsay, the occasional inconsistencies ... the work stands as the most reliable account of the Great Plague ... it has the truth of the conscientious and scrupulous historian, but its deeper truth belongs to the creative imagination."*

This makes good reading for psychiatric nurses: that it's not enough to worship the facts of mental illness without including how people communicate their distress. Of course if it's results you want, then plonk for randomised trials. However, everything hangs on what *counts* as results: what kinds of results. If you seek 'improvement results', then what kinds of improvement do you require and measured by whom? Objective outcomes may be straightforward enough when dealing with the problems cognitivists like to deal with, but what about the young man with low self-esteem because he's unable to engage with the opposite sex? Mary Midgley (2001, p. 147) puts the problem very well:

> *"There is no way in which we can collect facts about any significant aspect of human life without looking at them from some particular angle. We have to guide our selection by means of some value-judgement about what matters in it and what does not. And these judgements inevitably arise out of each inquirer's moral position."*

What then is the moral position of those who claim the title *nurse*? Is it to take the scientific high road that 'facts' are independent of morality and culture? Or does the title *nurse* entail a transcendent position wherein patients are engaged with at different levels and depths and including their experiences as part of what counts as evidence? It seems difficult to fathom a concept of 'nurse as scientist' whether pure or applied, and the dichotomy which nurses currently find themselves in – seeking to transcend medicine yet not professionally oppose it, espousing a different knowledge base yet still having to operate within practice areas largely defined by doctors – seems endless. Perhaps it's understandable when some psychiatric nurses wish to locate their work within a narrow scientism. Order, evidence, facts, measurement, accountability are everywhere and having to account for one's work outside measurable frameworks can be embarrassing. The attachment to measurable forms of interventions and the uptake of prescribing will consolidate scientific nursing within practice; the economic climate currently favours this and considerable efforts will be needed to sustain varieties of clinical practice.

> *"The best basis to substantiate clinical practice is the evidence of well-established clinical findings. Such evidence reflects verifiable, replicable facts and relationships that have been exposed to stringent scientific criteria."*

(Stuart 2001, p. 104)

However, I would argue that we should approach our work from a reflective, psychological position. Our investigations and the way we communicate with patients should be aligned with the humanities and avoid the parched nuances of medical treatment studies. Both of these views seek ascendancy and, in that sense, are discourse manipulations, as Foucault (1972) would have it, in that they both seek power. No doubt both are well intentioned and see themselves as placid and, ultimately, helpful. However, different implications for patients emit from both and cosy attempts to bring both positions together conveniently ignore this. Collapsing professional practice into vague assumptions of 'best things to all people' has not served nurses well in the past nor will it now. That said, professional suicide may be the price of a profession that can find no way around its 'jack of all trades' position. The RCT and all it implies seems hardly a way out of *nursing* whereas embracing the language, as well as the problems, of the common man might, albeit it at the cost of not rising above the common.

References

Ayer F 1936 Language, truth and logic. Gollancz, London

Bannister D 1998 The nonsense of effectiveness. Changes 16(3): 218–220

Burgess A 1978 A journal of the plague year: introduction. Penguin, Harmondsworth

Coleman R, Smith M 1997 Working with voices: victim to victor. Handsell Publications, Runcorn

Defoe D 1978 A journal of the plague year. Penguin, Harmondsworth

Durkheim E 1989 Suicide: a study in sociology. Routledge, London

Fisher R J 1993 Social desirability bias and the validity of indirect questioning. Journal of Consumer Research 20:303–315

Foucault M 1972 The archaeology of knowledge. Tavistock, London

Gournay K, Brooking J 1994 Community psychiatric nurses in primary health care. British Journal of Psychiatry 165:231–238

Hotopf M 2002 The pragmatic randomised control trial. Advances in Psychiatric Treatment 8:326–333

Jolley K, Bradley F, Sharp S 1998 Randomized control trial of follow up care in general practice of patients with myocardial infarction and angina. British Medical Journal 318(7185):706–711

Kierkegaard S 1941 Concluding unscientific postscript. Princeton University Press, Princeton

LaPierre R T 1934 Attitudes versus actions. Social Forces 13: 230–237

Loewenthal D 1999 Editorial: what is evidence and what is research? European Journal of Psychotherapy, Counselling and Health 2(1):248–250

Lowry D 1998 Issues of non-compliance in mental health. Journal of Advanced Nursing 28(2):280–287

Mair M 1998 Letter to editor. Changes 16(3):220

Malan D H 1995 Individual psychotherapy and the science of psychodynamics. Butterworth-Heinemann, Oxford

Martin J P 1984 Hospitals in trouble. Blackwell Science, Cambridge

Midgley M 2001 Science and poetry. Routledge, London

National Institute for Health and Clinical Excellence (NICE) (2006) Obsessive compulsive disorder: full guideline. Online. Available: http://www.nice.org.uk

Sackett D L, Rosenberg W M C, Gray J A M et al (1996) Evidence-based medicine: what it is and what it is not. British Medical Journal 312:71–72

Shakespeare W 1948 A midsummer night's dream. Penguin, Harmondsworth

Stanley N, Penhale B 1999 Institutional abuse: perspectives across the life course. Routledge, London

Stuart G 2001 Evidence-based psychiatric nursing practice: rhetoric or reality? Journal of the American Psychiatric Association 7(4): 103–111

Wiles R 1998 Patients' perceptions of their heart attack and recovery: the influence of epidemiological evidence and personal experience. Social Science and Medicine 46(11):1477–1486

3

Nursing research and the philosopher's stone

Shall we try reason? To my mind, nothing would be more sterile

(Michel Foucault 1982, p. 210)

THE QUALITATIVE–QUANTITATIVE DISTINCTION

An important preoccupation of nurses has been the nature of their research. Claims and counterclaims attend the worth of different approaches, and debates proceed against demands that nurses demonstrate an evidence base for their work. Although what counts as evidence is debatable, the view from the top is clear, the National Service Framework (DoH 1999) listing quantitative methods as ideal and with qualitative work coming way down the list.

- Type 1 Evidence: At least one good systematic review, including at least one randomised controlled trial (RCT).
- Type 2 Evidence: At least one good RCT.
- Type 3 Evidence: At least one well-designed intervention study, but without randomisation.
- Type 4 Evidence: At least one well-designed observational study.
- Type 5 Evidence: Expert opinion, including those of service users and carers.

Although qualitative studies are not ruled inadmissible, the above hierarchy explicitly prizes quantitative work and, ironically, at a time when psychiatric service user involvement is stated to be of growing importance.

For some, qualitative studies are mere collections of anecdotal, unverifiable data, a view typically bracketed with assertions that quantitative studies – particularly RCTs – are the 'gold standard' to which all else should aspire. However, while some qualitative studies also share this aspiration, utilising methods and concepts analogous to quantitative research, nursing is beyond that which RCTs can adequately investigate: much nursing is simply beyond scientific inquiry. This is contentious but it reflects my view (Clarke 1995) that qualitative research is a literary genre, its best examples expressing qualities found within fiction. In psychiatry, for example, many influential texts comprise fictional or other creative elements (Goffman 1960, Green 1986, Kesey 1973). In adult nursing also, narratives predominate and people's experiences, perceptions and attitudes are aggregated into a 'story' of what has happened or is happening to them. Such 'research' is hardly scientific, however, since its findings are poetically and not mathematically described. If we agreed with the 19th-century utilitarian Jeremy Bentham that 'poetry is no better than push-pin' we might consign qualitative research to literary dustbins and investigate only what is susceptible to quantitative measurement. In nursing, such investigations would probably cohere around drugs and their efficacy, or physical interventions and their outcomes. Internal meanings – the subjective experiences of nurses and patients – would have to be excluded since they are beyond objective representation. Yet it cannot be reasonable to exclude experience from research if the subjective worlds of patients and carers – whether professional or lay – are important.

However, although important, qualitative studies are often deficient in method. In fact, the issue is not so much their appropriateness in researching nursing but the problematic nature of how they are done. In particular, the manner by which qualitative researchers use data to generate theory rather than subject those data to rigorous analysis (irrespective of theory) is crucial. This creation of theory without evidence is exacerbated when the research is mediated by philosophical underpinnings that are predominantly continental. By continental is meant that way of philosophising that comes to us mainly – though not exclusively – through scholars from continental Europe (especially France) and whose ideas can be contrasted with British–American analytic philosophy which markedly differs. It is a contrast whose origins are eccentric to say the least.

ORIGINS

Simon Critchley (2001) recalls C. P. Snow's famous 1950s lecture where he denoted two distinct cultures among scholars that he respectively called 'the scientific' and 'the literary intellectual'. Noting that both groups had been educated to equal levels of sophistication he also observed that neither was on speaking terms with the other. That is, little if any theoretical or practical communication passed between them, nothing of productive value anyway. Snow – both scientist and novelist – was inclined to praise the scientists while castigating the literary intellectuals because of their non-involvement in real-world issues.

Whatever the degree of truth of this polarity, it continues to feature in contemporary philosophy with, on the one hand, British–American analytic (or objective) philosophy and, on the other, the more literary, quirky, fare that comes from the continent. British–American philosophy embraces the tenets of western empirical science, specifically the belief that deductive processes are how truth and validity are made known; it also uses the language of the real world. Not so continental philosophy with its solid fusions of history, literature and linguistics and the perplexing, sometimes dramatic, conclusions that these mergers produce. Often the result consists of difficult to follow, difficult to refute arguments that are wildly speculative, metaphysical and with Germanic vagueness added on. Not that any of this has precluded its influence on social, political and cultural discourses over the last 30 years. Nursing research, far from being immune to this, has careered towards it, remarkably so considering that nursing is a supposedly practice-based activity. Nursing theorists such as Patricia Benner (1994), for example, deploy continental ideas to reject any division between subject and object, a division which science – and analytic philosophy – holds dear. Benner, and nurse theorists generally, criticise anything that objectifies patients, insisting that nurses must now nurse *persons* and shun the distancing of patients occurring within systems of medical technology. In place of medical knowledge, nurses will acquire tacit 'knowledge' from experience, from practice. Tacit means 'implied but not expressed'. Implications, however, are hardly measurable; indeed that which is tacit is partly hidden and so open to multiple interpretations. And in a context of qualitative research, multiple interpretation is prized, the scientific view banished to sceptic's corner.

ANTIPATHY

A measure of the antipathy between both schools is that when the renowned French philosopher Jacques Derrida was nominated for an honorary doctorate by Cambridge University in 1992, established academics at the university opposed the move and forced a (rare) vote on it (which was lost). Putting matters bluntly, for some, the 'father' of continental philosophy, Martin Heidegger, is a genius; for others, his writings are gibberish. Certainly it's hard to deny the inherent woolliness and the density in continental writing or to see why it is often mistaken for profundity which, on close inspection, it isn't. What I object to is precisely this obscurantism which continental philosophy produces and which, in turn, acts as a smokescreen for poor investigative rigour. To make the point forcefully I need to acknowledge that qualitative research *can* be methodologically robust, for instance using multiple observers (Hinds et al 1990) to enhance reliability. Further, while RCTs might determine which treatments are best for, say, depression, they cannot determine if we should treat depression in the first place. To elucidate *that* means tapping into what depression is and the severity of how it is experienced by people. Putting this another way, qualitative research can challenge cherished assumptions about meaning and experience in health and illness; it can alter perceptions about what these are and suggest responses to them. However, elucidating meaning, cut adrift from any objective moorings, can produce the delusion that self is the only reality. Regrettable though this is, it starts from a respectable premise grounded both in the traditions of nursing as well as in its new-found attempts to redefine itself.

SUBJECTIVITY AND MEANING

Nurses seek to understand the meanings of their actions and qualitative researchers attempt to provide this. However, problems begin when they seek respectability for their work from the wider research community. To date, the commonest way of achieving this has been to force favourable comparisons between qualitative and quantitative approaches. This is complicated, however, because qualitative work, with its emphasis on verbal data and literary forms, doesn't have the numerical precision of its opposite number; actually it stands in deliberate opposition to numeracy and can even attack it as 'number crunching'. One way of boosting the reputation of qualitative research is to collapse its comparative claims into an equation whereby all research is alleged to be the same. In this way a truism takes hold, namely that 'science (too) is subjective'. As philosopher Rosalind Hursthouse (1978, p. 130) puts it:

> *"All those differences you used to think there were between poetry and science, or history and science – well, those differences don't exist. Scientists are human like the rest of us, and they can't keep their feelings, biases and prejudices, the influence of their age and environment, out of their science."*

But Hursthouse then denies that scientists are subjective in this sense. That scientists are personally involved in their investigations, for example in the selection and interpretation of data, is obvious but that they show the uneliminable involvement that the 'subjective' charge implies is untrue. Partly, the confusion stems from issues to do with the origins of knowledge as opposed to processes by which knowledge is investigated. Hypotheses emerge and are developed from whatever sources experimenters expose themselves to, true, but the investigative methods of science, of quantitative methods, are designed to prevent whatever subjectivity might unwittingly enter that which is to be investigated.

THE RCT

For example, scientists utilise procedures of sampling theory, data collection and analysis where data are 'reduced' to statistics so that levels (and implications) of significance can be worked out so as to facilitate *exact* replication. Facts are seen as external to individuals (although individuals may know them) and so conducive to rigorous testability aimed at disproving whatever hypotheses incited the research in the first place. As such, it is an approach that:

> *"does not yield eternal truth, but rather systematic doubt: rather than produce absolute knowledge it reduces uncertainty. And it can only answer questions of a factual nature."*

(Herbert 1990, p. 15)

In essence, the RCT seeks to disprove the outcomes it anticipates and comes unstuck in those cases where uncovered data increase the doubt by disproving the initial hypothesis. In contrast, qualitative research *accommodates* discordant data; new data which disprove or contradict existing categories simply have new conceptual or categorical significance conferred upon them. Such manoeuvrings diametrically oppose scientific principles, rooted, as they are, in a subjectivity whereby researchers can decide if verbal data merit new categorical significance or if they should be discarded.

FOUCAULT ET AL

The reiteration that 'science is subjective' is part of the appeal of continental philosophy and is especially celebrated in the work of Michel Foucault. An essential of that appeal is the insistence that psychiatry is an elite system (of knowledge) whose function is to enhance doctors' power. Further, it is held that psychiatric knowledge is but one of many truths; this, in turn, furthers the notion that 'practically any other type of knowledge is as valid as western science' (Glazer 2001). Such notions stem from Foucault's paranoia that everybody was out to get everybody, his insistence that grand narratives such as Marxism, psychoanalysis and history were discourses invented to service vested interests. Thus, the (supposed) altruism of the Victorians in building mental asylums was really about incarcerating those who were of little utility to capitalist expansion. As cottage industries begin to amalgamate and expand, so do they lose their familial capacity to protect those of their members unable to contribute to changing economic systems. On such readings, medicine constitutes a powerful clique that bends patients to its will: orthodox psychiatry, so it goes, being obstinately committed to treating mental illnesses as objective entities and with disgraceful disregard for patients' experiences.

Ultimately, what the continental critique seeks is an objective-free universe, an intellectual relativism where ideas do not account for (or enlighten us about) the world but are rather about acquiring power. According to Derrida, the end game is where we become '*liberated* from meaning' (Scruton 1996, p. 478) and free to interpret matters as we see fit, since interpretation is misinterpretation anyway. No text really states more than its own interests; to deny this, as I am doing here, is to believe (erroneously) that things *can* be disproved. Any belief of mine that this book is more than self-aggrandisement is a delusion. The point is this: am I wrong in thinking that this is the kind of 'philosophising' that drives most qualitative research today? Recently, while examining a PhD thesis, I was coolly informed by its writer – a fan of Foucault and Derrida – that its conclusions were what they were, its truths equal to whatever my (examiner's) responses might be to them! Such a view – that the self is the only knowable thing – is not easy to refute. But it is surely irrational to deny the existence of *some* correspondence between what is perceived and that which exists. In this case, doesn't the examiner bring to bear on the PhD his experience of academia at a level and depth which equip and empower him to do this? If not, if all truths are equal, how can we reach any decent consensus about right and wrong, morally or otherwise?

SHIFTING GAZE

The godfather of continental philosophy is Michel Foucault and the reader is referred back to my introductory notes on him. His influence on Benner's (and many other) nursing models and philosophies is obvious. At first sight, these nursing models seem liberating but they may actually be retrogressive. How? Well, Foucault's description (1973) of a shift in 'the medical gaze' advanced the notion that 18th-century medicine altered its focus from the person: 'what is the matter with you?' to the body: 'where does it hurt?' For Foucault, this quantum leap was the harbinger of that depersonalisation which came to characterise psychiatric practice and it is this assertion that renders him the most quoted philosopher in qualitative research. Today, medicine's gaze penetrates even deeper and, occasionally, Foucault's worst fears are realised. I recall, for instance, a claim by a miner with pneumoconiosis for compensation to the (then) National Coal Board being rejected by its Chief Medical Officer with the riposte that 'indeed pneumoconiosis was not a disease: rather was it a radiological picture'. In other words, it was not what the person claimed – an illness – but rather an invention of medical technology. Yet despite such criticisms, belittling advances in medical practice or questioning its scientific assumptions is still problematic. Such objections operate along a continuum but occasionally they assume anti-scientific postures tantamount to denying reality. Glazer (2001) relates how American nurses, influenced by Foucault, risked patients' lives with 'new age' interventions that had no rational basis at all. Hard to imagine in Britain, perhaps, although the psychiatric nurses' tendency to connect with the social, spiritual and psychological lives of patients at the expense of the bio-physical aspects of their illnesses can appear decidedly odd.

MORALITY

Foucault's writings gathered pace from the political unrest of the 1960s and, especially, emergent anti-psychiatric and feminist 'movements' with their alternative discourses on history, sociology and politics. In the case of social sciences, greater emphasis was being placed on the emotional aspects of people's lives. In Foucault's view (1982) the part of people most relevant to morality is feelings. This compromises western philosophy since the latter had always accorded to moral life a distinct rational component. What the emphasis on feelings now represented was less a concern with probity or truth and more a deliverance from social order and its restrictions. Thus, in the rise of professionalised helping the emphasis on self is not always convincingly demarcated from self-interest. Dalrymple's (1995) male patient, who savagely beat his girlfriend because 'she was doin' me head in Doctor', is an apt example of an 'ethic' that seeks to explain evil by appealing to feelings. What opposes this is social order and its institutions, invariably the pet hates of Foucault and his disciples. Marshall Berman (1983) notes the relish with which Foucault embalms people within institutions. Prisons and hospitals, for instance, are named and shamed as malevolent entities with people interminably trapped within them. Berman also notes (1983, p. 34) the sadistic teasing by which Foucault toys with readers:

> *"Do we think we feel a spontaneous rush of sexual desire? We are merely being moved by the 'modern technologies of power that take life as their object.' Do we act politically, overthrow tyrannies, make revolutions ... establish and protect human rights?"*

The answer is always 'no' because such activities are just appeals to authority, 'discourses on power' from which no revelation can come. Everything is discourse because the discourse is itself subject to discourse and on and on and on and on. But if Foucault contends that no truths exist other than as shadows of power interests within successive epochs, that nothing binds us to an authoritative past, then his is a risky undertaking for as Roger Scruton (1996, p. 6) says: 'A writer who says there are no truths, or that all truth is merely relative, is asking you not to believe him. So don't'.

SCIENCE HAS SHOWN?

Of course the rot had set in with Martin Heidegger (1962) who asks us to believe that there lies beyond beings (us) something called *Being* but that being of this world is one sure way of never being able to come to terms with it. To gain acquaintance with Being, we must take leave of this world, in the sense of abandoning objectivity. The problem with this is that the only thought and language we have is what we have. Since these cannot provide access to the outside (world), we clearly need a language that can. Working that out is what gives us the acknowledged density of Heidegerrian writing; entering that labyrinth is dicey for anyone not privy to the truths it contains.

> *"On the side of continental philosophy, a greater and greater cult of paradox and obscurity, an appetite which feeds on what it consumes and, as with a galloping illness, hardly allows the imagination to conceive its end: who can outdo Heidegger?"*

(Gellner 1959, p. 258)

Well, Foucault can, with his denial of the subject as having an objective entity – humans are fictions existing only in the texts which create them. For example, 'truths' evolving within (the growing number of) hermeneutic PhDs are not objectively verifiable. Indeed with qualitative research generally it becomes difficult to apply any objective yardstick by which to evaluate its findings. This can result in research that fails to connect meaningfully with practical nursing while concentrating on dodgy assertions about science and the improbability of reality.

ABSTRACTING DATA

A classic example of such assertions is contained in Sokal & Bricmont's (1998) account of continental philosophers abstracting data from physics and astronomy so as to further their claims. Essentially, these abstractions involve using material from subatomic physics so as to justify contentions about the supposed relativity of truth, time and existence. Nurse researchers have quickly picked up on this, their favourite manoeuvre being to employ Heisenberg's Uncertainty Principle to show that matter is not governed by laws of 'cause and effect'. In fact, this principle pertains only to *some* subatomic 'behaviours' and is irrelevant to most real-world scientific inquiries. Yet Heisenberg's Principle is depicted as analogous to social disequilibrium; without justification, subatomic uncertainties are alleged to characterise the entire scientific agenda:

> *"as a discourse involving the same kinds of rhetorical strategies, literary tropes, and unstable meanings as other forms of writing."*

> (Collini 1993, p. 1)

While it is wrong to regard scientific inquiry as *utterly* unimpeded by culture, it is nevertheless a gross distortion to claim equanimity between jumping atoms and a busy A&E department. Of course, we must equally guard against scientific claims to absolute truth or the tendency of some scientists to browbeat non-quantifiable methods. That said, qualitative researchers who set out to debunk scientific achievements do themselves little favour. Rather should they celebrate their values as non-scientific investigators whose work is less about method and more about the origins of knowledge and its social/cultural meanings.

NO POINT OF REFERENCE

Tricking out research which has no point of reference rejects moral frameworks as well as rationality: it represents the death of objectivity. Says Roger Scruton (1996, p. 479):

"that the subject is a fiction is itself a fiction, part of the attempt to claim over the objective world the kind of absolute sovereignty that attaches to a purely subjective view of things."

This subjectivity requires eliminating language as it is commonly understood: that is, questions need not refer to what has gone before. Hence, (tacit) nursing knowledge is not 'learning on the job' – a concept on which time and tradition has conferred some substance – but is now an elusive domain whereby experiential learning is imbued with deep significance. Indeed, continental philosophy is at its most pernicious when infusing ordinariness with seriousness or making each thing analogous to something else. It thrives on uncertainty, making converts not only of the genuinely undecided but of those in love with undecidability anyway. Ackroyd (2002, p. 72) says that for people who lose their nerve:

"What could be more attractive than a fearfully rigid and complex set of instructions on how to read and how to write?"

Paradoxically, those commandments flow from a philosophical rigidity which insists on constant and uncritical replication of disorder, of uncertainty, of manufactured profundity and the trivialisation of language. A. C. Grayling (2006, p. 228) pulls no punches:

"a cheap form of philosophy done by waving banners with Derrida and Heidegger on them, resulting in salaried logorrhoea, a thick stream of indecipherable nonsense that has spewed, like outflow from a mains sewer, into an intellectually polluted sea of fertility."

What began as a protest about overarching designs and professional exclusivity has itself become doctrinaire in its defiance of self-doubt and outside censure. Thomas Cahill (1995, p. 59) notes that when civilisations grow weary they lose confidence and he quotes Sir Kenneth Clark thus:

"Civilisation ... requires confidence – confidence in the society in which one lives, belief in its philosophy, belief in laws, and confidence in one's own mental powers."

Some qualitative nurse researchers will stay within recognisable reference points, tying their observations into solid reflections on nursing practice. While not science, they will uncover narratives and events that may push their practice forward. This will require a re-uptake of confidence about what psychiatric nursing is and what it seeks to do. From that will flow research strategies grounded in the problems of practice and delivered in idioms that readers will comprehend. However, this is insufficient for some, who, more and more, will adorn their inquiries with a philosophy of 'anything goes', examining odd questions in odd ways and with a language that would put the jabberwocky to shame.

References

Ackroyd P 2002 The collection. Vintage, London

Benner P 1994 Interpretive phenomenology: embodiment, caring, and ethics in health and illness. Sage, London

Berman M 1983 All that is solid melts into air. Verso, London

Cahill T 1995 How the Irish saved civilisation. Sceptre Books, London

Clarke L 1995 Nursing research: science, visions and telling stories. Journal of Advanced Nursing 21:584–593

Collini S 1993 The two cultures. Canto Edition, Cambridge

Critchley S 2001 Continental philosophy: a very short introduction. Oxford University Press, Oxford

Dalrymple T 1995 Don't bite the doctors. The Sunday Times, News Section, November 12th, p. 3

Department of Health 1999 The national service framework for mental health service. HMSO, London

Foucault M 1973 The birth of the clinic: an archaeology of medical perception. Tavistock, London

Foucault M 1982 On the genealogy of ethics. In: Dreyfus H, Rabinow P (eds) Michel Foucault: beyond structuralism and hermeneutics. Harvester, London

Gellner E 1959 Words and things: an examination of, and an attack on, linguistic philosophy. Routledge, London

Glazer S 2001 Therapeutic touch and postmodernism in nursing. Nursing Philosophy 2(3):196–202

Goffman E 1960 Asylums. Penguin, Harmondsworth

Grayling A C 2006 The heart of things. Phoenix Books, London

Green H 1986 I never promised you a rose garden. Pan, London

Heidegger M 1962 Being and time. SCM Press, London

Herbert M 1990 Planning a research project: a guide for practitioners and trainees in the helping professions. Cassell, London

Hinds P S, Scandrett-Hibden S, McAuley L S 1990 Further assessment of a method to estimate reliability and validity of qualitative research findings. Journal of Advanced Nursing 15:430–435

Hursthouse R 1978 Introduction to philosophy: an arts foundation course. Unit 13. The Open University Press, Milton Keynes

Kesey K 1973 One flew over the cuckoo's nest. Picador, London

Scruton R 1996 Modern philosophy: an introduction and survey. Mandarin, London

Sokal A, Bricmont J 1998 Intellectual impostures. Profile Books, London

4

On the literary character of qualitative designs: using diaries in psychiatric research

Only good girls keep diaries
Bad girls don't have the time

(Tallulah Bankhead 1903–1968)

THE MODERN WORLD'S FIRST DIARY

Thomas Cahill (1995) informs us that St. Augustine, when writing his Confessions, deployed a sensibility that is now so second nature as to make us forget the seismic shift that resulted from its first reading. For, in his Confessions, Augustine becomes 'the first human being to say "I" in the sense that we nowadays take "I" to mean'. Before Augustine, what we take to be private sentiment or revelation was curiously impersonal and static. Augustine initiates, through his writings, a level of psychological disclosure that is startling. Although, these days, blasé 'tell all' diaries and 'blow-by-blow' accounts of the (in)famous are common, nothing matches Augustine's depth of contemplation and his 'clear, poignant and ruthless' prose. He worms his imagination into literature such that personal narrative becomes the inherent agency of fiction. Augustine's is the first diary, the inaugural address of 'the self'. Whether such texts are written for personal salvation or for the edification of others will be the central preoccupation of this chapter.

WHAT ARE DIARIES: WHAT ARE THEY FOR?

The Shorter Oxford English Dictionary (1982) defines diary as:

> *"A daily record of events or transactions, a journal; specifically, a daily record of matters affecting the writer personally."*

The word 'personally' matters since most people recognise the innate privacy of diaries, the way they appeal to secrecy, intimacy, rehearsal of private thoughts, notes from the underground. And what are diaries for? Well, according to Aitken (1944, p. 8):

> *"If one should desire to know what life was like a hundred years ago, one could scarcely do better than make a study of the contemporary diarists."*

This is true but only up to a point: it overlooks the waywardness of diaries, their idiosyncrasies. Blythe (1991, p. 1) brings out these qualities:

> *"[diaries] are clearly the result of a form of pleasure-seeking, or of a passion for secrecy, some are records of the inner life, a lot are outlets for gossip and tale-telling, some are confessionals and some, by their faithfulness to the humdrum, are major historical documents."*

Again, the 'personal' assumes relevance in the way that diaries count as truthful accounts of what they purport to represent. What can be taken as 'truth' lies at the heart of any literature claiming to represent reality. In the case of qualitative research, claims to truth are also subject to reservation since they too stem from subjective sources. As such, in addition to examining the personal and/or public intentions of diaries, I will also explore the role of fiction in qualitative research and especially the capacity of diaries to account for the beliefs, experiences, perceptions and attitudes of their subjects.

THE HISTORY OF DIARIES

Diaries begin to become significant around the 17th century (the diary of Samuel Pepys, famously). The latter, while an indispensable record of its times, is also a private document since it is a) written in (easily deciphered) code, but b) revealing – with relentless charm and unselfconsciousness – the intimacies of Pepys' private life. Fanny Burney's (1940) diary also records its times while noticeably displaying many of the gifts of the novelist, a feature that occurs in diaries repeatedly. More recently, the diaries of 'Chips' Channon

(1967) recounted the fables and follies of the 1930s English 'Establishment'. Today's fashion is for 'reveal all' diaries seemingly begun by Peter Hall (1983) and while, before, diaries were often published posthumously, these days publishing one's reminiscences can be a positive career move and with readable, gossipy, witty, bitchy accounts *de rigueur*. Alan Clark's (1993, 1996, 2001) diaries fall into this vein, acerbically noting the highs and lows of comrade politicians but, as well, divulging the moral dubiety of his own behaviour. Clark was given to calling his diaries a 'work of art' and this implies a certain poetic licence, probably in support of readability and controversy. Such poetic licence, however, questions whether diaries, or any literary form, can count as viable research accounts. Like novelists, qualitative researchers come to their inquiries through naturalistic processes. For example, accidents of current biography infuse research activities and:

> "... as sociologists, we make problematic in our research, matters that are problematic in our lives. In fact, much of the best work in sociology ... is probably grounded in the remote and/or current biographies of its creators."

(Lofland & Lofland 1984, p. 8)

In other words, biography lifts research above the humdrum, rendering it meaningful, readable and exciting!

CRITICS

Personalising academic work is not without its critics, however. David Starkey (1997), for one, challenges the academic propriety of 'personal accounts', suggesting that scholars refocus to a more modest, detached anonymity. This, of course, supposes that detached objectivity is possible. The fact is, all history is written in the present; the past is an interpretation. In today's academic climate few assert complete objectivity; most concede degrees of personal involvement with their material. That said, some recent writers – called revisionists – have taken more than the usual liberties, making grand interpretations not so much from evidence as from a determination to impose meaning on to their data. Andrew Scull, a noted historian of psychiatry, reflects this tendency. Scull ploughs intentions into history: in *Museums of Madness* (1979), malevolent forces labour to exclude pauper-lunatics from 19th-century society, driving them into the all-purpose cauldrons that become the Victorian lunatic asylums. Other historians (Jones 1993, p. 67) challenge this view and, currently, a 'post-revisionism' (see Digby & Stewart 1996, Porter 2003) seeks to qualify the insights of scholars such as Scull (1979) and Foucault (2003) by setting their work within contexts of what *can* be known objectively.

An outrageous instance of interpretative excess was David Irving's (1997) account of the Nuremberg Trials where he gave credence to pro-Nazi accounts of the Holocaust. Norman Stone (1997) accused Irving of 'stretching the data' so as to fit his warped – if superficially well-researched – theories (and, indeed, Irving would lose his libel action against Deborah Lipstadt at the London High Court in March 2000: Lipstadt had accused Irving of 'holocaust denial'. Later, an Austrian court would imprison Irving for three years for the same crime (Elkins 2006, pp. 4–5)). Yet, Stone insists that *some* room be left for refining dominant accounts. The question turns on how much should rest on factual evidence, how to strike a balance between evidence and interpretation. Personal accounts do explicate past and present, yet issues of accuracy remain problematic and it needs remembering that the accuracy of qualitative accounts can even match the physical sciences.

That said, imagine what modern historians would give for a glimpse into the diary of any significant figure from the past. Turning this on its head, where would we be without Samuel Pepys' diary (1970) or Anne Frank's (1947) or Francis Kilvert's (1960)? None of these possesses replicability; none is the product of any methodology other than a desire to tell their story. What they do share, however, is an intensity and quirkiness that is part and parcel of narrative work, of personal reminiscence of self and others. Challenging their factuality doesn't demean their authenticity as perspectives of their times and surroundings.

DEGREES OF PERSONAL

In 1993 Alan Clark published his diaries to immediate acclaim. The intimacy of the material, its 'revelations', gave furtive pleasure to millions as it teased and 'sent up' its high-profile subjects. Watching someone poke their nose in others' affairs is irresistibly entertaining and Clark was good at it. He was especially clever at making his audience 'read between the lines', eliciting nuances of what he might or might not be revealing. Less effective, because overly laden with (eavesdropped) drawing room trivia, was Woodrow Wyatt's 1985 effort, a blancmange of titbits that failed to entertain because it was too self-serving, whinging and point scoring. Much more is needed than revelation – a certain style is required; malice, yes, but with the tongue firmly placed in the cheek. Joe Orton's diary (Lahr 1978) provided this with its eye-opening portrayals of 'the swinging sixties'. It had a staccato, epigrammatic style akin to the effect of flicking through a photo album; snapshots of a fast, frenetic life. Taking matters further, Roy Strong's diaries (1997) appeared to glorify indiscretion:

> *"exposing the mannerisms, squabbles, fashionableness, or lack of it, of the royal family, society and the art world."*

(Vickers 1997, p. 3)

Ken Tynan's (2001) diary similarly pushed indiscretion into more difficult, disturbing areas. Courting humiliation, his writhing images of physical, psychological and pecuniary misery became rather hard to bear. Why he disclosed what he did is perplexing: he had a tendency to shock, that much is known, or perhaps worsening illness tempered this and he simply wanted to post an honest account. What remains, however, is the dilemma of distinguishing the private from the verifiable and, while this matters little in avowedly fictional works, it does matter when events are paraded as having happened.

LIES, CONFIDENCE TRICKS AND MIRRORS

The novelist Andrew Sinclair is adamant that Kingsley Amis lied in a story where Amis (1992, pp. 220–221) has Sinclair, a Scot, sponge drinks from him in a bar. The story occurs in Amis' *Memoirs* where he admits at one point (p. 306):

> *"Many times in these pages I have put in people's mouths approximations to what they said, what they might well have said, what they said at another time, and a few almost outright inventions."*

We can defend such inventions if they make psychological and/or artistic points. In such cases, we trust that the diarist is an artist obligated to veracity. However, where the tendency is to employ outright fiction, it becomes difficult to discern what kinds of truth are being presented. Not that readers fail to bring their own perspectives to bear on what they read even if diaries have a way of sucking their readers in.

Blythe (1991, p. 1) puts it thus:

> *"a diary is a kind of looking glass. At first it reflects the diarist. But it ends by revealing the reader."*

This requires literary skill. Eschewing mere recitation of 'facts', the diarist engages with readers creatively and entertainingly. For example, Defoe's *A Journal of the Plague Year* (1978) is as important to the development of the novel as it is a historical account. While often grounded in fact (it deploys statistics, for instance) it also contains fictional elements; we don't, for example, know whether all its characters are real. Thus did Anthony Burgess (1978, p. 6) call it 'a confidence trick of the imagination, a rather cunning work of art'. Yet diaries are not novels: how can they be when their content is tied to the diarist's interests? The novelist, alternatively, cannot but allow characters a certain 'freedom'. There are real differences at play here. For example, in respect of Roy Strong's diaries, Hugo Vickers (1997, p. 3) opined that Strong:

> *"has behaved badly in publishing private confidences and he probably knows it."*

Naming names grounds you because it entices readers into believing that 'this is how it is'. The novelist, however, creates more space, through characterisation, for distancing, camouflaging, going deep. Harking back to Amis' *Memoirs* (1992) it may be that, as a novelist, he could not adjust to a non-fictional form and so depicted characters in – to them at any rate – an uneasy light; diaries are apt to disturb their subjects. In my case, publishing diary material (Clarke 1996) that showed conflict among forensic nursing teams led to accusations of violation of autonomy and self-respect. Shocked that I had portrayed them as conflict ridden, these forensic nurses accused me of underhandedness, of killing the truth. Perhaps I had but if novels come from how experience is interpreted, is not this true for diaries as well or for qualitative research generally? After all, what differentiates them other than the levels of fiction they deploy?

THIN DISGUISES

Perhaps changing the names might alter the ethics. Would labelling one's reminiscences as fiction redefine their status? The radicalism of the 1960s fermented this question, inciting writers to produce books that challenged normative concepts of fiction. For example, Capote coined the term 'faction' to describe his novel *In Cold Blood* (1966) where he interspersed actual people and events with invented dialogue. Capote later accused Normal Mailer of stealing the form for his 1968 account of Vietnam War protests, *The Armies of the Night* (1968), although Mailer subsequently declared that such writing abandoned responsibility for creative fiction. Well, it depends on the thinness of the disguise; the distinction between fact and fiction can be dazzlingly obscure. Capote could have avoided the charge of unethical behaviour had the characters in his 'faction' not been real people. In fact, his book was received ecstatically by critics and public alike and was enormously influential on how novels were subsequently written. Reading chapter six of Julian Barnes' *Flaubert's Parrot* (1984) – winner of the Booker Prize for Fiction – one constantly reminds oneself that it *is* a novel and not non-fiction.

Sometimes the reverse is the case and fiction is used to augment factual accounts. In *The Female Malady* (1987), Elaine Showalter critically reviews the radical psychiatry of R. D. Laing from a feminist perspective. For Kotowicz (1997, p. 103), her book was little more than 'a concoction of insinuation, rampant prejudice and distortion of fact' derived from fictionalised sources. However, while Showalter does rely on fiction, it is the fiction of women's experience of mental distress. A more striking example of the genre is Clancy Sigal's novel *Zone of the Interior* (1976) which completely fictionalises the radical psychiatry of 1960s England. Its main protagonist, Dr Willie Last, is an irreverent, Scottish, pot-smoking, radical psychiatrist and very reminiscent of R. D. Laing. Although Laing is mentioned in the book *as Laing*, Laing rightly saw that he was Last and successfully fought the book's publication in Britain (Laing 1994) (the book was finally published in 2006). Yet, although transparent in its method, Sigal's novel throws light on issues barely touched on by more objective biographies of Laing (Burston 1996, Clay 1996, Kotowicz 1997). Speaking from its own time, its account of 1960s psychiatry becomes a compelling artefact of 'what happened', as well as being the best first-hand account of psychiatric nursing from the same period.

FACT AND FICTION

Fergal Keane provided an interesting take on the balance between what is observed and the subjectivity of the observer. In the 1997 *BBC Huw Wheldon Memorial Lecture* (Keane 1997) Keane spoke about the 'art' of reporting 'the news'. In this, he appeared to conflate 'facts' and 'truth', the implication being that facts cannot speak for themselves. Gill (1997) retorted that this only served to confuse and possibly even distort matters. However, achieving a clear-cut objectivity is a contested notion and contingent on what it means to 'know'. Claims to objectivity are asserted to depend on quantifiable data; observe, for instance, Sagan's (1997, p. 23) defence of 'the scientific method':

> *"If you know a thing only qualitatively, you know it no more than vaguely. If you know it quantitatively – grasping some numerical measure that distinguishes it from an infinite number of other possibilities – you are beginning to know it deeply. You comprehend something of its beauty and you gain access to its power and the understanding it provides."*

Qualitative practitioners, however, insist that numerical supremacy is a myth and that personal accounts add perspective and depth to understandings of people and events. This is true but misses the point that quantitative knowledge operates outside of perspective, refuses to be brought within any perspective but its own. While, generally, we need perspective as a means of insight into ambiguous and tendentious relationships (and particularly so in mental health) there is no denying that both kinds of knowledge sit uneasily together, their proponents constructing markedly different frameworks of what counts as mental illness and how it should be responded to.

HEALTH CARE

In psychiatry, texts are composed of two sorts: first, there are compendium-style volumes which marshal facts, figures and clinical data; second, there are accounts (Barnes & Berke 1971, Jamison 1996, Millett 1991) which describe things in personal terms. The latter are often more informative – and readable! – than the former. Indeed, psychiatry needs a personal discourse inasmuch as patients' stories are not just of symbolic value, they have therapeutic significance in that they can change how care is organised and delivered (Launer 2002). Nolan (1993) and Gittins (1998) have charted psychiatric nursing history through nurses' (and patients') oral accounts as well as through student nurses' diaries and 'reflective journals' (Landeen et al 1995, Taylor 2005) which also yield valuable data. Burman's review (1995) revealed how successful diaries are in gathering data on acute illnesses and 'minor symptoms'. However, they were less successful in accounting for major life crises, chronic illness or infrequent episodes of illness. Various writers have commented on the level of complexity of what needs recording: the simpler the data, the easier the task. So that using diaries in psychiatry will be problematic due to such things as stigma, violence, social sanctions and the often volatile nature of interactive care and therapy. Not for nothing have health-care diaries been restricted to logging symptoms and rarely venturing into experience. That said, a small number have done this.

Katherine Mansfield's (1928) chronicle of her last illness is an example as is Barbellion's (1920) similar account. Mary Barnes' (Barnes & Berke 1971) parable of madness and regression is also notable as is Kate Millett's (1991) journey through Irish psychiatry, the latter a more frightening account than any academic text could provide.

GOING ELECTRONIC

In 2002, Paty reported that diaries were now used in almost 25% of clinical trials. This surprisingly large figure resulted from the inclusion of electronic as well as written systems to monitor 'medical moments', recordings of such items as migraine attacks or changes in mobility.

Electronic diaries had actually materialised on the Internet in 1995 and today run to tens of thousands, forming a virtual community of diarists. It might be thought that this development heralded a radical departure from orthodox diary keeping. But as Sorapure (2003, p. 2) points out:

> "the insistent present-ness of the web ... parallels the diary's traditionally non-retrospective written form."

Indeed, with the Internet, diaries move even closer to the perimeters of 'experience', seemingly shutting down divisions between what is private and public. This produces questions of access as well as problems of accountability. It also means that the e-mail tendency to write instantly – unlike with pen and ink – blocks reflection and appraisal of what is written or how. For whatever else one can say of e-mail, it's done us no service in respect of grammar, syntax or spelling. More so does it drive an appalling confusion between what is information and what is knowledge.

BIAS

In Oppenheim's (1966, p. 215) view:

> "the respondent's interest in filling up the diary will cause him to modify the behaviour we wish him to record. If, for instance, he is completing a diary of his television-viewing, this may cause him to indulge in 'duty viewing' in order to have something to record, or he may view better types of programmes to create a more favourable impression."

Therefore, it is likely that subjects might choose particular events, writing them up in ways that suggest therapeutic engagement and so displaying themselves in a good light. That is, the diarist, knowing that they will be read, writes their diary with that in mind. Unable to smother their fascination at being found out, generations of adolescents have lived in masochistic 'dread' lest their 'anyone reading this will die' diaries will be discovered, their secrets revealed. All diarists are proto-exhibitionists eager to be 'caught in the act', their private thoughts exposed. Oscar Wilde knew this: in *The Importance of Being Earnest* (Wilde 2003, Act 2, p. 27), Algernon asks Cecily 'Do you really keep a diary? I'd give anything to look at it. May I?' to which Cecily replies: 'Oh no! You see it is simply a very young girl's record of her own thoughts and impressions, and consequently meant for publication'.

Well, it's maybe a bit more complicated than that. For if diarists are about the business of reporting life then their capacity to withhold themselves becomes a pivotal consideration. Blythe (1991, p. 32) quotes Thomas Jones (1870–1955) on this point:

> *"A diary, by hypothesis, forbids complete self-effacement, but I hope that I have also steered reasonably clear of self-glorification, the vice of this sort of book."*

Compiled without thought of being read, diaries circumvent bias but this rarely happens and is, indeed, psychologically implausible. Your average diarist wants to be caught in the act, their trousers firmly down!

CAVEAT

The Sunday Times discovered a diary (Mega 1997) which disclosed that a former moderator of the Church of Scotland – a one-time mentor to Prime Minister Blair – had been a lifelong paedophile. The author of the diary having died, its contents reached *The Sunday Times* through a family member. It seems that this *is* an example of a diary left without intention of publication. Yet, if so, why was it written? Why wasn't it destroyed? Something of the aforesaid desire to be exposed? Perhaps a compulsion to let the truth become known? A yearning for self-mortification or punishment? Or just one further cynical act of aggression?

Latham & Matthews (1970, p. xix), responding to the frankness in Pepys' diary, say that they 'were of their nature private: Pepys kept them entirely for his own enjoyment'. Well, if so, why did he take the trouble to protect them during the fire of London? Similarly, centuries later, 'Chips' Channon buried his diaries in a churchyard to protect them from the Blitz. Naturally these diarists wanted their thoughts read; within a context of 'whiff of secrecy', no doubt, but read nevertheless.

CONCLUSION

What fascinates about diarists is what Blythe (1991) calls their dedication to ordinariness, their eagerness to record the minutiae of life. Perhaps the capacity to infuse ordinariness with noticeability is a gift. Certainly, the persuasive diaries are the ones that communicate readably and movingly. Doubtless, it is overly romantic to suppose that research diaries could stand comparison with the personal kind. We have conceded that the diarist's art is essentially private and composed of what is real and what is imagined. So how do research diarists immunise themselves against fictional intrusions; what are the mechanisms of immunity? Is it indeed something they should do?

There probably is room for structured diaries in health care, recording aspects of personal illness as an aid to therapy, for instance, or using them to focus upon a defined topic or event(s). In this, the diarist's role is to describe anew his subject's propensities for happiness, pain or whatever, conveying the warp and weave of events and people.

I believe that diaries operate between novels and biography, roughly between fact and fiction. But I am hard put to define how 'facts', in the hands of any writer, acquire fictionless status. We have become used to statements which assert the subjective/creative elements in biography and history. We hardly blink at 'the novel' which sets out to solve scientific questions – *Fermat's Last Theorem* (Aczel 1997) – or elaborate on medieval philosophy – *The Name of the Rose* (Eco 1983) – or discuss war, madness and therapy (Barker 1992). Should we be surprised, therefore, if diaries become the research method par excellence in qualitative research, with their inimitable capacity to chronicle intimacy, privacy and the vicissitudes of life? Of course such research cannot claim the sobriquet 'science' but then neither can the 10 000 works of fiction that are of inestimable value to our wellbeing.

References

Aczel A D 1997 Fermat's last theorem. Viking, London
Aitken F 1944 English diaries of the XIX century 1800–1850. Pelican, Harmondsworth
Amis K 1992 Memoirs. Penguin, London
Barbellion W N P 1920 A last diary. Chatto, London
Barker P 1992 Regeneration. Penguin, London
Barnes J 1984 Flaubert's parrot. Jonathan Cape, London

Barnes M, Berke J 1971 Two accounts of a journey through madness. Free Association Books, London

Blythe R 1991 The Penguin book of diaries. Penguin, Harmondsworth

Burgess A 1978 A journal of the plague year: introduction. Penguin, Harmondsworth

Burman M 1995 Health diaries in nursing research and practice. Image 27(2):147–152

Burney F 1940 The diary of Fanny Burney. Dent, London

Burston D 1996 The wing of madness: the life and work of R D Laing. Harvard University Press, Cambridge, Massachusetts

Cahill T 1995 How the Irish saved civilisation. Sceptre Books, London

Capote T 1966 In cold blood. Hamilton, London

Channon H 1967 The diaries of Sir Henry Channon (edited by Robert Rhodes J). Weidenfeld & Nicolson, London

Clark A 1993 Diaries. Weidenfeld & Nicolson, London

Clark A 1996 The Alan Clark diaries. Phoenix, London

Clark A 2001 Diaries: into politics. Phoenix, London

Clarke L 1996 Participant observation in a secure unit: care, conflict and control. Nursing Times Research 1(6):431–440

Clay J 1996 R D Laing: a biography. Sceptre Books, London

Defoe D 1978 A journal of the plague year. Penguin, Harmondsworth

Digby A, Stewart J 1996 Gender, health and welfare. Routledge, London

Eco U 1983 The name of the rose. Secker & Warburg, London

Elkins R 2006 Three years jail in Austria for holocaust denial. The Independent, February 21st, pp. 4–5

Foucault M 2003 The birth of the clinic. Routledge, London

Frank A 1947 The diary of Anne Frank. Hutchinson, London

Gill A A 1997 The truth about fish fingers. The Sunday Times, Culture, October 26th, p. 34

Gittins D 1998 Madness in its place: narratives of Severalls Hospital 1913–1997. Routledge, London

Hall P 1983 Peter Hall's diaries: the story of a dramatic battle (edited by Goodwin J). Hamilton, London

Irving D 1997 Nuremberg: the last battle. Focal Point Publications, London

Jamison K R 1996 An unquiet mind: a memoir of moods and madness. Picador, London

Jones K 1993 Asylums and after. Athlone, London

Keane F 1997 The 1997 BBC Huw Wheldon memorial lecture. BBC 2, October 20th

Kilvert F 1960 Kilvert's diary. Cape, London

Kotowicz Z 1997 R D Laing and the paths of anti-psychiatry. Routledge, London

Lahr J 1978 Prick up your ears: the biography of Joe Orton. Allen Lane, London

Laing A 1994 R D Laing: a biography. Peter Owen, London

Laing R D 1960 The divided self. Penguin, Harmondsworth

Landeen J, Byrne C, Brown B 1995 Exploring the lived experiences of psychiatric nursing students through self-reflective journals. Journal of Advanced Nursing 21(5):876–885

Latham R, Matthews W 1970 The diary of Samuel Pepys: a new and complete transcription. G Bell, London

Launer J M N 2002 Narrative-based primary care: a practical guide. Radcliffe Medical Press, Abingdon

Lofland J, Lofland L H 1984 Analyzing social settings: a guide to qualitative observation and analysis. Wadsworth Publishing Company, California

Mailer N 1968 The armies of the night. Weidenfeld, London

Mansfield K 1928 The journal of Katherine Mansfield. Constable, London

Mega M 1997 Blair's school mentor was sex abuser. The Sunday Times, News Section, May 25th, p. 7

Millett K 1991 The looney bin trip. Virago, London

Nolan P 1993 A history of mental health nursing. Chapman & Hall, London

Oppenheim A N 1966 Questionnaire design and attitude measurement. Heinemann, London

Paty J 2002 What is a subject diary and how do regulations apply? Applied Clinical Trials, September 1st, pp. 38–43

Pepys S 1970 The diary of Samuel Pepys: a new and complete transcription (edited by Latham R & Matthews W). G Bell, London

Porter R 2003 Flesh in an age of reason. Allen Lane, London

Sagan C 1997 Billions and billions. Headline Book Publishing, London

Scull A 1979 Museums of madness. Allen Lane, London

Shorter Oxford English Dictionary 1982 Clarendon Press, London

Showalter E 1987 The female malady. Virago, London

Sigal C 1976 Zone of the interior. Thomas Y Crowell, New York

Sorapure M 2003 Screening moments, scrolling lives: diary writing on the web. Biography 26(1):1–23

Starkey D 1997 Studies self-love of the new dons. The Sunday Times, News Review, June 1st, p. 9

Stone N 1997 Flawed judgements. The Sunday Times, Books Section, February 23rd, p. 1

Strong R 1997 The Roy Strong diaries 1967–1987. Phoenix, London

Taylor B J 2005 Reflective practice: a guide for nurses and midwives. Open University Press, Maidenhead

Tynan K 2001 The diaries of Kenneth Tynan (edited by Lahr J). Bloomsbury, London

Vickers H 1997 The Roy Strong diaries 1967–1987. Book Review. The Sunday Times, Book Section, May 11th, pp. 1–3

Wilde O 2003 The importance of being earnest and other plays. Modern Library, New York

Wyatt W 1985 Confessions of an optimist. Collins, London

Can there be a nursing ethics?

SECTION CONTENTS

5

The rights of the case: the Rosie Purves story

Judge not, that ye be not judged

(Matthew vii, i)

'I KNOW MY RIGHTS'

The refrain 'I know my rights' is relatively new but it carries great rhetorical force. We are now a rights culture; women's rights, gay rights, animal rights, children's rights, fathers' rights, the list is endless. It wasn't always like this; until recently moral philosophy took the form of asking 'what was the right thing to do'. Today, much ethical thinking – as understood by a politically savvy and better informed public – consists of notions of rights, how to acquire them but, more so, what to do if they are thwarted. When setting out those qualities which constituted being English, Jeremy Paxman (1999, p. 22) put 'I know my rights' at the top. However, although rights are frequently seen as inalienable, often the basis for their 'rightness' is simply that they are asserted. What the asserters overlook, however, is that rights impose obligations on others for their satisfaction. If I have a right to something, then, by implication, someone else is going to have to satisfy it. Indeed, the more one looks at rights – and their satisfaction – the more one agrees with the philosopher Jeremy Bentham that rights are 'nonsense: nonsense on stilts'.

HEALTH CARE

An examination of a specific claim will reveal what Bentham meant; for example, you might think that within socialised medicine you possess rights to health care. However, someone with private health insurance might claim a greater right and, given finite supplies of care, is likely to jump the queue and/or acquire better services. You could argue that you each have equal moral rights to what is available and, all things being equal, this is hard to deny. But in working through what actually happens, the privately insured person will get their due, else why pay privately in the first place? So, demanding rights is one thing, having them met is another.

An important question is whether humans are *intrinsic* bearers of rights or if rights exist independently of claims to them. According to Roger Scruton (1995, p. 198) some rights stem from nature and not from social convention. For example, there are:

> *"natural rights to life and limb, and to the freedom that is presupposed in the exercise of choice. There is also a natural right to property."*

In fact, formidable criticisms can be made of claims to natural rights. Horner & Westacott (2000, p. 162), for example, point out that those who claim individual freedom and property as if they were 'natural rights' are, in truth, expressing political preferences rather than timeless truths. However, for now, I wish to examine how *expressing* rights affects those to whom they are directed and how professionals, in particular, respond to rights claims. Clearly, claiming a right requires the satisfaction of something that is of value to the claimant, something that has precedence over whatever might inhibit its satisfaction. This last point will become central to Rosie's case later on.

CURRENT PREOCCUPATIONS

These days we take rights very seriously indeed. We are generally better informed as well as being more litigiously minded – the walls of my local A&E department display advertisements for law firms for those who may have slipped on someone else's floor. Today, too, professionals are aware of the need to comply with clients' demands even if only to disarm their anger or prevent them 'making a scene'. In many cases, we have come to believe that demands are synonymous with rights but they are rarely this as we saw in the case of competing claims to health care. Should we defend this principle of private ownership or should the state distribute money and goods in equal measure? Initially, it seems just for governments to do this and, actually, they do distribute wealth to an extent as well as placing restrictions on its use. But if participation in private health schemes is property owning (and it is) and given that it is government sanctioned, can we really talk of equitable rights to health care? When Bentham said that claiming rights was nonsense he, of course, meant natural rights, the claim to rights as inalienable and not legally provided for: but without such provision, most of us will find that claiming rights is pretty meaningless. Take the ownership of land: Scruton (1995) argues that by mixing his labour with an object – tilling the land – the worker makes the land his own, he acquires rights to it. However, such a view disenfranchises nearly every major landowner in Britain whose ownership stems from having arrived *after* the initial tilling, hanging the tiller, and then taking the land as his due. And even when ownership is legally determined a local authority may compulsorily purchase it where the owner's only remaining right is getting a fair price for what is no longer his. That there exists a residual unfairness about such moves suggests that we like notions of rights and fair play and that we generally suspect those who encroach on these.

RIGHTS

A right can be about doing something (such as worshiping) when it is called an active right. A right might also be about having something (to be told the truth, to be looked after) and in such cases is called a passive right. There are also rights to be in a certain state, for instance to feel free or happy, or to take a certain attitude, for instance against government. We have rights to education, a living wage, free speech, privacy, trial by one's peers, right of way and right of appeal. Rights are things we can earn, enjoy, exercise, fight for. They can be recognised, infringed, abridged, protected; they can be moral, legal, religious, political, statutory, customary, constitutional, contractual or utilitarian. You have a right to receive calls for assistance but this imposes obligations and duties on the claimers since they can hardly exempt themselves from the same right.

Do we have a right to act without interference from others? Probably not. I do not have rights to your property for example; or do I? After all, don't I rightfully take a portion of your taxes when I collect my social security payments? However, we probably accede to this when voting for political parties who inform us, in advance, that they will do this. What if you did not accede to it? This cropped up recently when Jonathan Miller (2003) insisted on not paying his BBC licence which he called 'a tax on television'. Miller believed that the legality of the licence had lapsed due to what he called the 'digital cornucopia' whereby television was now a multiple channel industry. Miller's question is why can't he be *asked* to pay, and says if he was that he probably would. He also highlights that most prosecutions are against people on benefits who cannot pay; for those who can, he notes that some of the licence money will find its way into the expense accounts of BBC executives.

NO RIGHTS AT ALL

Some things we do not have rights to: to success or failure, for example. Nor do we have rights to perceive, ache, itch or injure, unless, with the latter, we are licensed by the state, as an executioner or in war. Indeed, the interplay between rights, justice and law throws up some curious contradictions. When British courts sentenced three gay masochists to prison terms of three and four years, the prisoners appealed to the European Court of Human Rights at Strasbourg. These men had caused 'bodily harm and wounding' to each other but had mutually consented to this in private. They claimed the British were violating their privacy and were supported in this by the British civil rights group Liberty. According to Liberty's Director John Wadham:

> *"It's utterly ridiculous that the sexual activities of a few consenting adults in private should be illegal, when it's nobody's business but their own."*

(Ames 1997)

Professor of Law, David Feldman, was of the view that:

> *"The interest in allowing people to express their sexuality ... is not less important than the interest in allowing people to pursue sports. Sport is fun, but sex for many people is more than fun: it is a form of self expression."*

(ReviseF65)

Although the injuries inflicted were severe, the court papers state that 'permanent injury or the need for medical attention' did not occur. However, the European Court ruled against them stating: 'the determination of a tolerable level of harm where the victim consented was primarily a matter for the state authorities' and that such interference was directed at 'the protection of health and morals' (Spanner Trust 1997). Lawyers for the men pointed to uncensored activities such as boxing and tattooing, both painful, destructive but consensual and, of course, ultimately, there is the question of the courts punishing *them* without *their* consent! In British law Lord Templeman's view was that: 'society is entitled and bound to protect itself against a cult of violence'. However, good law ought not to rely on personal preference; there need to be more specific outlines of what is or is not acceptable. To say that the law should mind its own business challenges how far you would allow private behaviour to go. Could these men, for example, have used violence that would have required medical intervention? If yes, to what degree? Could someone, for instance, consent to have themselves killed so as to further their own or another's sexual pleasure? Or what happens if things 'get out of hand' and inadvertently 'go too far': who becomes culpable? Wadham's defence of 'privacy' is a red herring; a range of things, such as non-consensual sex, makes privacy irrelevant. The central element is consent but even here, as I've suggested, matters are not straightforward either and are certainly not so in mental health contexts.

THE HIGHEST MORAL GOOD

What is the highest moral good? It's a good question. One could respond in different ways but it seems that justice is as high a good as you can get. What is considered just, of course, impacts on rights and the part they play in determining what is just. According to Plato, to see justice clearly is to watch it operate in the workings of the state and its structures. Harmony within a state does not depend on whether its subgroups are co-equal as much as the extent to which they complement each other. Although reason is the final arbiter of what counts as just, its expression must not injure the overall functioning of the state. This emphasis is also present in the empirical philosophy of David Hume. Here, regard for justice doesn't rest on other people; rather, it comes from approving systems that construct rules, obedience to which is in a public interest. It follows that obedience might not be in our own interest but rather serve the greater good. For example, entering a social contract involves forfeiting that which might benefit me. I consent to this so that society functions in reasonable harmony. However, as noted, the balance between individual and community can be contentious. Does government, for instance, have the right to compel me to do military service? Should trade unions compel us to join them and pay subscriptions when we don't want to? Why should the BBC have the right to force me to pay a licence fee if I don't watch its programmes? Why shouldn't I have the right to smack my kids *as I see fit* and without the social contract of EEC membership and its rules getting in the way? These are the issues of justice and rights that currently make the headlines; resolving them requires working through the relative interests and outcomes for all concerned but, as well, the extent to which this is informed by legal provision.

In some cases, though, legal provision may not be required. Jeremy Paxman (1999, p. 118) points out that a comparable word for privacy does not exist in French or Italian while in England privacy is a fundamental principle. Paxman initially thinks it curious that no law enshrines this principle but then considers that:

> *"constitutional protection is only necessary in a society in which it is presumed that the individual is subsidiary to the state."*

Since a principle of privacy lies at the heart of 'what it means to be British' as well as the formulation of its laws, Paxman concludes that an actual privacy law is not required. Well, possibly not as protection from state intervention (at least not yet). However, in an age of computerisation and micro-storage, with their burgeoning stores of information about us, who knows what legislation may be needed to protect us from the future gaze of government agencies.

HEALTH CARE

This is the rights background against which we must examine questions of health-care provision. Relationships with patients, for example, are now more complicated in respect of growing concerns about ethics. In the age of the 'Patient's Charter' medical power has been curtailed particularly where questions of rights are involved. In Rosie's case the question is whether someone has a right to care from nurses *of her choice*. The answer depends on what is just and the way in which rights impose obligations on others even when, in this instance, the content of the 'right' is morally repugnant.

ROSIE PURVES

Rosie Purves has been a paediatric staff nurse for almost 30 years. Ask her why and she replies:

> *"I've always loved my job. There has never been anything else I wanted to do. I love working with children. It is where I thought I could serve people best."*

(*Nursing Times* 2004, p. 24)

However, throughout that 30 years she had remained conscious of her black skin and of the need, as she saw it, to work harder, to be better, to achieve more, in order to win acceptance. This state of mind, she believed, was normal and only recently had she (and other black colleagues) begun to recognise that such beliefs were not right. In May 2004, Rosie Purves was awarded £20 000 – the highest possible payout – when she won a race discrimination case against her employer. An employment tribunal ruled that Southampton University Hospital NHS Trust had been 'effectively silent and complicit' in the racist demands they had made upon her and in the name of servicing a patient's demands. Here is what happened.

POWER AND ABUSE IN ORGANISATIONS

The racism began when a consultant paediatrician informed Rosie that a mother did not want her to look after her six-month-old child, recently admitted to Rosie's ward with cystic fibrosis. The mother had said that although happy with the care Rosie was giving, she – the mother – was racist and objected to further care from a black person. The mother said this was 'her right'. The consultant took pains to inform Rosie that this was not his view but that the care of the child was paramount.

Thoroughly ashamed, Rosie felt unable to tell anyone.

"I was distraught, but nurses don't argue with consultants."

(Davies 2004, p. 3)

While the team on the unit told her that they did not see her as black they nevertheless participated in removing the child from Rosie's care. These arrangements persisted through several hospital admissions for a period of over a year and acquired something of the quality of an open secret. Each time the child was admitted, its mother would request its removal to the side of the ward where Rosie didn't work.

"I felt alone, I thought everyone was colluding with the mother to keep themselves safe. I felt that by moving the baby the other staff were sending out the message that it was OK to be racist."

(*Nursing Times* 2004, p. 24)

The racism ceased in 1997 but when the child was re-admitted in 2000 it began again with increased vigour because, by now, two mothers were involved, the second of whom began to verbally abuse Rosie.

*"Don't go anywhere near my f*king child. I don't want people like you looking after my child and that is my right."*

(*Nursing Times* 2004, p. 24)

For seven years – until transferred to another hospital – the child's mother and her friends referred to Nurse Purves as 'Black Rosie'.

They made racist phone calls to her and taunted her with comments about 'black jelly babies'. For several years, Rosie had to use a back entrance to the hospital in an attempt to avoid her tormentors.

WHAT HAPPENED NEXT?

The case becomes more complex. Rosie also worked in a special needs school where a sister of the first racist was a pupil. When racist abuse began here as well, the school's head took decisive action against the abusers. However, such action was not forthcoming within Rosie's NHS trust and it needed the intervention of a trade union to instigate an employment tribunal. The tribunal concluded that the NHS trust had been 'silently complicit' in the racism and made its award. Rosie declared herself 'relieved about the verdict'. However:

> "Racist abuse ruined my life. If I could put the clock back I would put my pride aside and speak up. Verbal abuse needs to be tackled. As nurses we accept patient anxiety, but we don't have to put up with abuse – not verbal, not racist, not any form of abuse."

> (Nursing Times 2004, p. 25)

Although Rosie remained magnanimous towards the racist mother, dismissing her as 'too ignorant to know better', she is caustic about how the mother's views were permitted. From the hospital's point of view, they unreservedly apologised to Rosie; they have also stated that no one will go through the same ordeal. Following the tribunal's decision, a spokeswoman for Southampton University Hospital NHS Trust stated that Rosie Purves was 'a superb nurse' stating that it was:

> "committed to ensuring that no one will ever have to go through the same ordeal."

> (Davies 2004, p. 3)

FACTS AND FIGURES

Before looking at the issue of refusing nursing care, we can clarify matters by looking at some facts from a recent survey (Crouch 2004). In this survey, 22% of white nurses reported the likelihood of their ethnicity exposing them to verbal abuse whereas 81% and 77% respectively of black and Asian nurses reported likewise. On the question of offering nursing care to racists, 8% of black nurses said they would withhold it whereas 53% stated that racism would force them to look for work elsewhere. These cold statistics are perhaps less shocking: they fail to convey the full horror of what can actually take place. Staines (2006, p. 12) lists the widely reported case of racist nurse Christine Mitchelson who, according to Nursing & Midwifery Council (NMC) case notes, used words such as 'darkies', 'wogs', 'chinkies', 'slanty-eyed' and 'black bastards'. Staff nurse Grant Uttley informed a Caribbean patient who had had Caribbean food: 'You don't want that shit'. He was given a caution. Staines also reports that 30% of racist bullying came from colleagues but that 45% was by managers and senior personnel. Findings also suggest that this may be the tip of a covert iceberg and that much of racism is institutionalised into processes of job selection and promotion. In an interview with Chris Hart (a nurse consultant) Crouch (2004, p. 24) also discovered the extent of racism in the NHS. According to Hart:

> *"Black nurses are the target of overt and conscious racism. It's a huge issue in inner city areas where there are increasing numbers of nurses from overseas."*

In other words, there is an (alleged) racism in our city hospitals of which Rosie's case is but a visible example. Rosie herself believes this to be the case. Matters are not helped by the absence of policies to deal with racism; surveys of racism suggest that NHS victims talk of phoning their husbands, wives, families, as Rosie did, in order to relieve the stress. The assumption seems to be that, in the NHS, racism goes with the territory. Well, if true, then dealing with it should also go with the territory. At least we could identify the factors that permitted an organised, persistent, racism to be directed at a nurse who was trying to do her best.

THE RIGHTS AND WRONGS

'I know my rights' shouts the racist mother. Does she have such rights? Clearly *she* thinks she does. She may not see herself as racist of course; witness a recent statement directed at asylum seekers, to wit: 'I have nothing against them: I just wish the government would send them back where they came from'. However, ignorance is not bliss, it is base, and we have to reckon how this woman's racism contaminated a treatment setting, humiliating one if its members, while shaming the rest.

Was there any justification to the demand that the child receive white nursing? Or did the tribunal get it spot on when damning what had occurred as 'silent complicity' with racism? Few, apart from racists, would disagree with this surely. Nevertheless, the 'rights' of the racist mother were met and the racism reinforced. What options did they have? Most might agree that under no circumstances should the child have received white-only nursing. That said, withholding treatment is problematic: the child has done no wrong and can hardly be penalised for its mother's behaviour. However, Rosie had done nothing wrong either – she hadn't done anything – yet her defencelessness and vulnerability were hugely exploited.

CULTURE

In such matters, compromise usually plays too great a part in how things are done. Trying to do right by most people significantly informs social and political encounters in English life. According to Paxman (1999, p. 138) English people believe in:

> *"a common sense middle way, in which as much as possible is left to individual discretion. One of the reasons the English have never been much interested in either fascism or communism is that they have a very sensible scepticism about what the state can achieve."*

Allied to this distrust is the principle of privacy and, although the English are extremely good at building institutions, they retain a faith in 'minding one's own business'. No doubt, too, power and inequality of position play their part, as Rosie herself found out: 'you have to think twice before going up against a consultant'. So, given the conditions, what would or should have been the right thing to do?

Could the child, for instance, have been made a ward of court with the mother prevented from further intrusions into its treatment? This may incense those who value the sanctity of parent–child relationships. However, rights and justice have to be weighted. Mention has been made of Plato's idea of balance between the subgroups that constitute society and of how the intolerable may need to be tolerated if this ensures stability.

However, in contemporary Britain, sustaining inequalities between people because of race or ethnicity is morally objectionable and the sheer obnoxiousness of racism now outweighs *any* considerations of unity or balance. So also should moral principle provoke recourse to law where this is possible. Yet the law that could have prevented the mother from entering the ward and thus protected Rosie from racial harassment was not utilised. Equally, could legislation have been invoked to ensure that the child receives care albeit separately from its mother? It therefore remains an open question as to why no legal redress was sought for Rosie and/or the child. But it also casts a difficult light upon the trust's statement that, in similar circumstances, treatment and care will be denied.

THE HEART OF HUMANITY

We may not expect that governments will strive to achieve excellence on our behalf but we surely have a right to expect them to legislate to protect our fundamental values. Racism strikes at the heart of humanity; in these cases discriminated-against nurses were frequently terrified and forced into seeking professional help. Racism can be comparatively easy to manage, for instance when it is overt rather than furtive (jokes, for instance, are a particularly nasty form of racism because typically spewed out as inoffensive: 'it's *only* a joke', or 'what! haven't you got a sense of humour?', see Ch. 12) or where it is rationalised as being for the greater good, in this case the priority accorded to the child. Further, racism is especially virulent when downplayed as 'something else'. For instance, focussing on verbal abuse of all nurses (for instance in A&E departments) implies that this is of the same ilk as racism. However, black and Asian nurses contend with a *consciousness* of discrimination that takes, as its first premise, beliefs about inherent inferiority. When one's racial subgroup is threatened, one senses one's ethnicity as more coherent, more solid and, from a defensive viewpoint, necessarily so. And while some would prefer these matters to be addressed in heterogeneous, multi-racial, multi-ethnic terms, this diminishes the fundamental baseness of black and Asian discrimination. The NHS should establish mechanisms to deal with all types of prejudice, of course, but there is a special need to respond to black and Asian racial prejudice. It may be that black nurses need to organise along the lines of the American National Black Nurses Association Inc., established over 30 years ago to represent the interests of patients as well as nurses within health systems. Admittedly, anti-racist legislation is tougher in Britain than in the United States and the Commission for Racial Equality already exists to identify abuses. Well, perhaps, except that, in the case of Rosie Purves, the Commission was nowhere to be seen.

ALL FIRED UP

There is no question that the notion of rights 'fires people up' and we appear to be less concerned today with what is the right thing to do – what it is to be a good person – and more preoccupied with obtaining things and becoming petulant when we don't get them. Staking a claim to something assumes overall agreement that what is being claimed is just, that it is normative. However, some will persist in their demands even when suspecting that just conditions do not apply. Few racists can be unaware of the distaste they incite in others; thus, may their resoluteness be attributable to compounds of irrational hatred, the knowledge that their demands 'work', that there exist, somewhere, silent wells of approval or, at least, indifference?

Although racism and stupidity are not necessary bedfellows, ironically Rosie bore her persecutor no ill will largely because she saw her as 'ignorant'. According to the ancient Greeks, inability to reason is the chief characteristic of intemperate people, an inability to see right from wrong. Yet racists may be extremely knowing about the consequences of their actions and sly in bringing about trouble and strife. We have to oppose this although working out what to do is never easy. One stumbling block is that what constitutes a right does not always correspond to what *is* right. For example, the right to press freedom permits the dissemination of pornography which is distasteful albeit not as distasteful as censorship. Equally, in these cases must we balance individual proclivities against the general good. For example, we can buy health care over and above what NHS patients can normally expect. We can, in Mrs Thatcher's (in)famous utterance, get the doctor we want, where we want, at a time we want and so on – provided we pay. Also, we don't seem bothered by the provision of women's hospitals nor that some families object to their relatives being intimately nursed by staff of the opposite sex or of their relatives being housed in unisex facilities. So it does seem that patients have rights about who nurses them and where and when. However, how far can this be extended and in what directions? Most health providers would defend a right to female nursing where there exists an aversion to males whether on religious or other grounds. Expectant women, for instance, are entitled to female midwifery although few exercise it, most objections to male midwives coming from husbands and partners! So that where agreement exists that something is good or desirable, then claiming it as a right may be seen as just. The claimant will be on much stronger grounds though if legal statute protects the right and/or prescribes the conditions of its exercise and, indeed, Rosie's case was won on grounds of violating the Race Relations Act (1976). However, it was moral outrage which put this Act on the statute book to begin with and which ultimately compelled its application in Rosie's favour.

LEGAL PROVISION

'England is a nation thickly planted with laws' (Bolt 1980) and most rights have some basis in law. However, the general picture is patchy and inconsistent. Few would deny equal rights for women. However, the specifics of its provisions – such as rights to maternity leave – have to be legislated for and governments keep a watchful eye on what they grant or withhold. Now that Britain has ratified the European Convention on Human Rights, fewer of its citizens will seek redress at Strasbourg unless domestic courts rule against them. Although appeals to the European Court – established in 1950 – were initially few, since 1980 cases are running at approximately 14 000 a year. It is unlikely that Rosie Purves would have derived satisfaction from the European Court since this court has been particularly conservative on race rulings. The wording of Article 14 which covers race is vague but more so has the court tended to defer to the respective countries of its jurisdiction before making decisions. That said, a more robust consensus on racism is emerging within Europe and undoubtedly the court's rulings will become stronger. Having said this, sufficient British law exists to deal with these matters and we may hope for its more rigorous application in future.

Finally, it says something for the much vaunted autonomy of the nursing profession that it couldn't come to Rosie's defence. Although the essence of the case is its racism, the events also intimate a subterranean culture where, despite the ferocious rhetoric of nursing professionalisation – including a much vaunted Code of Conduct – little shift has actually occurred in the hegemonic power of medics. With more than 170 000 black and ethnic employees – about 13% of the workforce – the NHS remains dominated by white staff in its upper echelons. Recent innovations, such as the 'Breaking Through' initiative (Paton 2005), are designed to move black and minority groups into higher, managerial positions and this may lead to positive change. However, racial vigilance needs to permeate the entire arena of health care if something as dreadful as the discrimination against Rosie Purves is never to happen again.

POSTSCRIPT

Following the case, Rosie was assured by Southampton University Hospital NHS Trust of an independent review into racism. However, Rosie informed *Nursing Times* (2006, p. 2):

> *"They told me because of financial problems they weren't going to do that. After the tribunal an awful lot of nurses have had the*

courage to come forward and talk to me about problems. There is still a problem and Southampton has done absolutely nothing."

When asked about this by the *Nursing Times* (2006, p. 2) a spokesperson for the trust stated that a meeting had been held with Rosie Purvis [*sic*] and that an equal opportunity and diversity group would be set up with Rosie as one of its members. It may be worth noting that the NMC – four years after its inception – does not have an equality and diversity strategy, has no records of trends relating to racism and has never in its history – as NMC, ENB or GNC – taken formal note of the ethnicity or racial background of its members. It has, however, announced an *intention* to remedy much of this.

References

Ames P 1997 Online. Available: http://www.jhu.edu/~newslett/02-21-97/News/Sado-masochists_face_jail_abroad.html

Bolt R 1980 A man for all seasons. Heinemann, London

Crouch D 2004 Colourful language. Nursing Times 100(39):24

Davies B 2004 Exposed: racist shame of NHS. Daily Mirror, May 18th, p. 4

Horner C, Westacott E 2000 Thinking through philosophy: an introduction. Cambridge University Press, Cambridge

Miller J 2003 I may be standing in the dock but it is the BBC that is on trial. Daily Telegraph, July 16th, p. 7

Nursing Times 2004 Racist abuse ruined my life. Nursing Times 100(32):24–25

Nursing Times 2006 Trust reneges on race review pledge. Nursing Times 102(10):2

Paton N 2005 Breaking down racial barriers. Nursing Times 101(5): 26–27

Paxman J 1999 The English: a portrait of a people. Penguin, London

Race Relations Act 1996 HMSO, London

ReviseF65. Online. Available: http://www.revisef65.org

Scruton R 1995 A short history of modern philosophy, 2nd edn. Routledge, London

Spanner Trust 1997 Text of European Court of Human Rights judgement in the Spanner Case. Online. Available: http://www.spannertrust.org/documents/Eurofinal.asp

Staines R 2006 Is racism a problem in nursing? Nursing Times 102(10):12–13

6

Outrageous protocol: on the question of control and restraint

The rotten apple injures its neighbour

It is sometimes the case that those who succeed in life do not like to be reminded of their humble origins. This applies to individuals but also to one's group, be this a professional grouping like nursing or a more diffuse gathering such as the nation state. So it was that when Brian Abel-Smith published his seminal *A History of the Nursing Profession* (1977) it annoyed those who believed that nursing had originated with the 19th-century Protestant deaconesses at Kaisersworth – who had influenced Florence Nightingale – or the Catholic Sisters of Mercy whose enduring image suggested selflessness, idealism and devotion. What Abel-Smith revealed was that the origins of Nightingale nursing lay with the characters we encounter in Charles Dickens' novels, for example Mrs Gamp, whose embodiment of her profession is smelling of gin. A woman of perspicacity, she spread herself wide in the service of others and was thus needful of some comfort in order to do so. As Dickens (1951, Ch. 19) tells it:

> *"The face of Mrs Gamp – the nose in particular – was somewhat red and swollen, and it was difficult to enjoy her society without becoming conscious of a smell of spirits."*

In Charlotte Bronte's *Jane Eyre* (1946) a madwoman is looked after by Grace Poole who doubles her wages by keeping her ward a secret as she performs the difficult business of containing her 'in the attic'.

These are the first nurses: either confined with their charges in privately maintained attics – for those who could afford this – or ministering to the sick and poor for the price of a gin. For the pauper lunatics of Victorian England the statutory requirement to build asylums must have been a welcome refuge for the thousands who quickly inhabited them. The worst imaginings of the Victorians were enshrined in these new asylums, their water towers ascending into the clouds like red brick skyscrapers. 'Castles of fantasy', Elizabeth Shoenberg (1980) called them, conjuring up bizarre notions about what went on inside them which was actually an evolving custodialism and punitiveness (Martin 1984). According to Gadsby (2005, p. 18):

> *"Traditionally the worlds of the asylum and the prison have been inextricably linked. They kept unwanted people at arm's length [serving] as a reminder of how close social exclusion is to us all."*

That custodial/punitive dimension finds expression not only in inpatient services that survive but also in the growth of forensic services from the 1970s. Yet, proclamations of a caring, holistic stance where social exclusion is exchanged for acceptance and where non-judgementalism extends to all has been a war-cry of modern psychiatric nursing. However, the success of this perspective has depended on a playing down of the custodial aspects of the job.

In *Madness and Murder* (2000), Peter Morrall contends that psychiatric nurses too easily dismiss public concerns about anti-social behaviour by mentally ill people, that they are blasé in refusing to assuage the moral panic that psychiatric violence provokes, especially its randomness and inexplicability. Morrall has a case here and no doubt the general public, concerned that not enough is being done to protect them, would see his point. However, matters of public concern can be taken out of proportion and portrayed as more terrifying than they really are. The tabloid press, for example, are ever ready to exaggerate whatever psychiatric deviance happens their way and they are helped in this by the fact that most people rely on them for their information and are often ill-informed by other sources.

CHRISTOPHER CLUNIS

Jeremy Laurance (2003) points to the case of Christopher Clunis as a turning point in the history of British psychiatric care. In December 1992 Clunis, diagnosed with schizophrenia, killed a man in the London underground. Several days prior to this he had been seen wandering the streets threatening people with a screwdriver and bread knife. The case alienated the public from a better understanding of the problems of mentally ill people in the community.

It increased apprehension about violence and it fostered doubts about how this could be effectively managed. Laurance notes that while compulsory admissions to hospital for 1990–1991 were of the order of 18 000, by 2000–2001, the year that Morrall's book was published, the figure had risen to 26 700. Over the same period, the number of forensic psychiatric beds had doubled reflecting a psychiatric system driven by fear as well as a collective ignorance. The solutions proposed by Laurance (2003) are premised on his perceived failure of community psychiatric policy; essentially, he argues that services remain overly skewed towards professional perspectives. Notwithstanding a fashionable rhetoric of consumerism, services are still insufficiently geared towards, or controlled by, those who use them. Says Laurance (2003, p. 89):

> *"The mental health services need to execute a 180 degree turn to face away from the professionals and towards the people with mental health problems. The patients not only have to take over the asylum, but all the services that lie outside it."*

For Laurance, services remain reluctant to allow patients some control of their treatments through negotiation with professionals. People should have a menu of what is available to them and which can be tailored to their specific needs. In essence, we need to rethink the provision of community psychiatry with participation of service users at planning, implementation and evaluation levels.

Of course, secure accommodation will still be required for offenders and responsible judgements made about people's potential for aggression and violence. However, increases in coercive detention and burgeoning forensic services are often energised by imagined acts of psychiatric aggression, fuelled by tabloid reactions. The most recent official figures available (Appleby 1999) for psychiatric violence do not support assertions about it being on the increase. Indeed, it is ironic that such figures are decreasing or at least remaining static, while those for criminality generally accelerate (Howitt 1998).

RESPONSE

However, Morrall's criticisms require a considered response. In general, while he is right about the broader picture, he misses important details. For example, although most psychiatric nurses work outside forensic systems, it has not proved difficult to staff them; nothing suggests that psychiatric nurses avoid this kind of work. Equally, the psychiatric nursing literature has failed to produce a critique of the new custodialism apart from some sniping at systems of control and restraint (C&R) which they spawned. Morrall (2000) correctly argues that psychiatric nurses should acknowledge the custodial aspect of their work but that they have never *formally* rejected this constitutes an implicit acceptance. The latter of course is clothed within a veneer of person centredness and holistic rhetoric and, indeed, some forensic units even claimed to be therapeutic communities. For example, my research in forensic units (Clarke 1999) exposed a conflict-ridden ambiance in which some nurses expressed distaste towards the obvious manifestations of custodialism while others embraced it freely. The nurses divided into two groups – controllers and carers – with neither in any mood to take criticism from the other; theirs was a mutual regard of modest loathing. And if any one entity accentuated the fractiousness it was the use of C&R to subdue patients. This procedure is the talisman of forensic psychiatric nursing, the single most important device that stands between them and institutional mayhem, or so they would have you believe.

CONTROL AND RESTRAINT

There is no universal method of implementing C&R. Developed within the prison service, it comprises a set of choreographed manoeuvres whereby a team of professionals incapacitates an individual with, it is argued, minimal physical and psychological stress. Not the least problematic aspect of C&R is the dearth of information about its use but, more so, the absence of knowledge about how it is experienced by those on the receiving end. Actually, discussions in the literature have concentrated on technique: should the 'face-down' approach be used; for how long should someone be restrained, and so on. There is something to be said for such discussions if C&R remains in use and it looks very much as though it will. For example, the independent inquiry into the case of David Bennett (2003), who died while 'under' C&R, did not call for its abolition, thus cementing its use both in general and in forensic practice. That said, the inquiry *did* call for modifications, for example restricting the length of time for which a person can be restricted and prohibiting the face-down approaches. My view is that these modifications are inadequate and that the psychological and physical safety of patients is only assured if C&R is abolished. Crucially, the Bennett Inquiry judged the NHS guilty of 'institutional racism' and I mention this because race is an aspect of C&R – as is gender – that is unerringly absent whenever mental health teams discuss its application. When discussions do occur, following individual instances of using C&R, the agenda is about ironing out procedural or technical problems that occurred during its use.

Some years ago, I spent several months as a participant observer in two forensic units. I was struck by the nurses' uncomplicated enthusiasm for C&R: almost all of them – apart from a small number of women – praised it and saw no ethical problems in its use. All were quick to paint a picture of impending chaos were it not available. Their contention was that, without it, staff would have to 'pile in' on disruptive patients and that such uncontrolled responses were more likely to cause injury. In the light of the David Bennett case we now know that this is not so and that, indeed, inflicting injuries on patients (and staff doing C&R training sessions) is fairly common. However, allowing that the accountability of those deploying C&R is weak, even approximate data on its physical or psychological consequences are hard to find either locally or nationally. What stood out in my study was the nurses' belief that, given the nature of forensic care, C&R had to be *necessarily* available to them.

Such beliefs feed into a self-fulfilling prophecy whereby the availability of C&R makes its implementation more likely. A comparison may make this clearer. In the United States, the easy availability of guns has made firearms, in and of themselves, an issue, their sheer accessibility a contributing factor in incidences of injuries and killings. Some deny this, stating that it is not guns that matter but their owners; in violent situations, they say, it matters not that guns are accessible, what matters is human intent. This sounds intuitively wrong and liberal/progressive American politicians have tried in vain to tighten gun laws and reduce the slaughter. My point is that the availability of something, be it handguns or C&R, makes its use more rather than less likely, that a consciousness of access creates a mindset that fixes on events in such a way that, in this instance, C&R becomes inevitable.

An example from my study (Clarke 1999) explicates this. Certain patients' behaviours seemed to get picked up and acted upon by some, especially male, nurses. For instance, if a patient remained in bed beyond a certain hour, a nurse would start in on him (or her) to get up and get dressed. Beginning with modest encouragements but quickly building to stern exhortations (to rise and shine) these encounters invariably provoked tension. Both arbitrary and uncalled for, these interventions had no basis in therapeutic policy or strategy, and they were common.

PATIENT AWARENESS

An intriguing question is this: to what extent are patients aware of the presence of C&R in their forensic units? During an interview with a psychologist in a London unit, I was informed that C&R had:

> *"increased the number of incidents. Without exception the nurses say that they think it's great. The punters know where these techniques come from."*

If so, one wonders what they think about carers who feel a need to engage in procedures that are aggressive, pain inducing and dehumanising. Gallon & McDonnel (2004) – one a director of nursing, the other a consultant psychologist – have presented evidence showing just how destructive, physically and psychologically, C&R can be, and Professor Gournay (2001, p. 22), referring to a UK Central Council for Nursing, Midwifery and Health Visiting (UKCC) commissioned report on managing violence (which he chaired), stated:

> *"The report team is of the unanimous opinion that the use of pain to obtain compliance is a breach of the patient's human rights and that this practice should be immediately abandoned."*

Several (especially female) patients have referred to the indignity of being subjected to this procedure. One woman said to me: 'they've found *another* way to hurt us' (Clarke 1988) while a second defined its role within forensic units as 'an arm behind the back and into the seclusion room situation' (Clarke 1991).

GENDER

According to May & Kelly (1982) nurses respond more sympathetically to patients deemed mentally ill, such as those with schizophrenia, and less so to those not seen as ill in quite the same way, for instance people with personality disorders. This finding is confirmed by Markham & Trower (2003) who say that nurses express more negativism towards patients with personality disorder than to those with depression or schizophrenia.

In respect of women with personality disorders being nursed by men, the situation becomes more complex. I, too (Clarke 1999), observed animosity towards patients with personality disorders which was exacerbated if the patients were women. It became clear that when implementing C&R some male nurses were sexually aroused when forcing young women to the floor. Given that these women had committed offences (or were believed capable of doing so) they could be perceived as 'bad girls' who, having been compulsorily admitted, had still not 'learned their lesson'. Ray Rowden (2003) points to a traditional neglect of women's welfare in secure units where they comprise about 10% of the patient population. Rowden relates that women complain of being routinely patronised by staff, often being referred to, and dealt with, as 'bad girls'. In Rowden's view, issues of sexuality are 'poorly understood' by forensic nurses: just as these services have been labelled 'institutionally racist', so there is inattention to questions of gender and maintaining women's dignity.

INSIDE THE BOX

When I raised the issue of sexuality and C&R on an Internet discussion list (Bowers 2006) reactions were varied but, occasionally, outraged. Most of the responses were from senior nurses in academic or service roles. Unsurprisingly, there occurred a peremptory demand that I produce 'the evidence'. For example, 'how big was my sample?', 'how chosen?', 'how can we assess the reliability and validity of your methods?' and 'the generalisability of your findings?' I felt that this attempt to shift matters to questions of research method was but a ploy to deflect attention from the topic. Some attempted to tackle the issue directly: one respondent focused on distinctions between thoughts and actions, conceding that we should not condemn 'the intrinsically human *potential* for sexual arousal in physiologically/emotionally charged situations'. Someone pointed to the undoubted stress involved for everyone involved in C&R but that it would still be regrettable for male nurses to respond in this way. One writer acknowledged that 'occasionally men might get aroused when restraining female patients' but insisted that this didn't imply anything about the profession overall. One male practitioner, who used C&R, asked: 'could not the same criticism be made against females restraining men?' Well, perhaps, although extant testimony implicates men alone. The following statements are from my research (Clarke 1991) and are intended to breach the denial that surrounds the topic. Discussing C&R, a female staff nurse typically responds:

> "*I mean women are quite prepared to do it but the men will push the women out of the way to do it, quite often.*"

To the suggestion that some might experience a 'turn on' during C&R another female nurse stated:

"Yeah. I think that's fundamental to quite a few people, even some of the therapists."

When asked if the turn on could be of a sexual nature, she replied:

"With some people there's an element of a sexual turn on, I think. I'm not saying that they would abuse that person. But I think that there is an element of that in it. I think, thinking back to when we had three psychopathic women, there was certainly something like that in some people. It's quite a powerful thing to hold somebody down."

These quotes carry the dangers inherent in any qualitative work (see Ch. 4). However, they represent a broad testimony from forensic units. In addition, the issue is not about sexual arousal as such but the inability of those involved to see outside the box (of C&R), to deal with C&R as more than a set of techniques that require fine tuning; for them to assume that wider issues of ethics and gender as well as normal relations apply within forensic units as much as anywhere else. And how outrageous that the ordinary decencies of everyday life do not apply, in this instance, to women patients? In everyday life, where physicality is a factor, women are normally attended to by women; for instance, most women would surely object to being 'frisked' by male security guards or police officers. Even nightclubs who employ 'bouncers' to check for drugs now station women as well as men at their entrances. Women police officers, specially trained, are customarily present when women are interviewed in cases of rape or alleged rape. Male customs officers are not required to perform intimate examinations in search of drugs or other contraband. Why, therefore, in psychiatric care, are male nurses empowered to degrade women by wrestling them to the ground, holding them down, immobilising their limbs, inflicting pain on them, in the name of C&R? If C&R is to be used on female patients, couldn't it at least be female nurses that do it? It is unacceptable that women be stripped of their dignity by male nurses seemingly unable to appreciate the complex moral and social issues that underpin concepts of personality disorder. To proceed as if this term *defines* who or what these women are, or any patient for that matter, is both reductive and wilful. Mills (2003) draws attention to how socially constructed distinctions between normal and abnormal are sometimes construed as madness and sanity, and she quotes McInnes (2001) that female patients, wanting respect, can be labelled 'borderline personality disorder', their 'demands' interpreted as antagonistic and aggressive. Finally, what is it about female psychiatric nurses that they acquiesce in procedures which define female patients as undeserving of the same gendered conditions that they themselves obtain in their everyday living?

MACHO CULTURE

Rowden (2003) characterised state hospital care as exemplifying a 'macho culture' and much of this has percolated into the regional and local forensic units which were set up following the recommendations of the Butler Report (1975). It was in one of these units that Mr Bennett was killed and while his death was not intended, there nevertheless was absent a commitment to ensure just and dignified standards of care. For the future, we need to ensure that the Bennett Inquiry recommendations are implemented. Above all, there should be a centrally managed accountability for the use of C&R.

In light of some of the inquiry's recommendations, implementing them will raise challenging issues. For example, the requirement that no patient be held in a prone position for more than three minutes raises more questions than it answers. What, for instance, happens when the three minutes is up and the patient is still excitable or aggressive? Answers to this do not come easily which is why they are persistently raised by supporters of C&R. Clearly if it transpires that three minutes is insufficient it may be asked: why bother with C&R at all? Hopefully, these issues may force a wider debate on how to de-escalate difficult situations and not allow them to fester and erupt. Part of the answer is, surely, a sea change in attitudes towards dangerousness and a pulling away from the custodial trap into which psychiatry – its doctors and nurses – has yet again fallen. Having created a forensic system which is restrictive, claustrophobic, full of apprehension and steeped in a consciousness of repression, why express dismay if its inhabitants become ever more aggressive.

Ideally, C&R should be banned. Had Mr Bennett been killed with an injected substance, that substance would now be withdrawn, its pharmaceutical manufacturer under sanction. Commenting on the Bennett Inquiry's recommendation to stop face-down restraint, Bradford (2004) stated that the procedure should continue but that staff should be trained not only in C&R but in cardiopulmonary resuscitation as well. That sounds ominous. Are we to countenance interventions whose likelihood of cardiac collapse is such that resuscitation trolleys have to be on standby? It really is something when a harebrained idea like this is spouted without irony or self-doubt. Yet it indicates the 'mad, bad and dangerous' mentality that infects the thinking of many psychiatric nurses. We have enjoined a coercive mentality, created a designer violence so as to immobilise the 'non-compliant' within custodial settings. I am informed that 'control and restraint' is now a misnomer, that its current euphemism is 'care and responsibility' (Shifrin 2005).

LAST POINTS

The Bennett Inquiry stated that C&R should be a last resort, should not involve pressure on the neck, thorax, abdomen, back or pelvis and should be used for the shortest time possible (Strachan-Bennett 2005). Significantly, it did not rule out inflicting pain or the use of mechanical restraints. Currently the National Institute for Mental Health is attempting to establish national accreditation for anyone working as 'trainers in violence' for health staff. Well, that's something I suppose. Standardisation is no doubt a good thing and will improve matters. However, the word 'standard' can also be taken to mean 'norm' and new rules, implicitly, become a sanction for the continuance of C&R. But why the need for violence by anyone? Why the obsession with dangerousness, absconding, malevolence and control?

STOP PRESS

In December 2006, the latest report by Professor Louis Appleby (2006) made headline news when its homicide figures were yet again seized upon by the tabloids. The report's publication aroused cynicism given that the government is to again push its mental health legislation, with compulsory powers, through Parliament following a very successful lobbying against the bill. Even as the report was being published, over 100 MPs signed an early day motion for a better bill. Appleby's dramatically large homicide figures also seemed at odds with those of Taylor & Gunn (1999) which had not indicated any great surge or increase. And even if taken at face value, Appleby's figures are less than those killed on our roads each year by speeding police cars in hot pursuit. Now there's a thought.

References

Abel-Smith B 1977 A history of the nursing profession. Heinemann, London

Appleby L 1999 Safer services: national inquiry into suicide and homicide by people with mental illness. Department of Health, London

Appleby L 2006 Avoidable deaths. Department of Health, London

Bowers L 2006 Discussion list manager. Online. Available: http://www. city.ac.uk/sonm/mhld/staff

Bradford S 2004 Face-down restraint is necessary. Nursing Standard (Letters section) 18(25):30

Bronte C 1946 Jane Eyre. Zodiac Press, London

Butler R A 1975 Report of the Committee on Mentally Abnormal Offenders. Home Office and DHSS, Cmnd 5698, London

Clarke L 1988 They've found another way to hurt us. Changes 6(2):54–56

Clarke L 1991 Therapeutic community practice within a secure environment. Unpublished PhD thesis. University of Brighton, Falmer

Clarke L 1999 Challenging ideas in psychiatric nursing. Routledge, London

Dickens C 1951 Martin Chuzzlewit. Oxford University Press, London

Gadsby A 2005 Opinion. Nursing Times 101(5):18

Gallon I, McDonnel A 2004 Issues around control and restraint training in the United Kingdom. Paper given at the 9th European Mental Health Nursing Conference at Jury's Hotel, Dublin, February 28th

Gournay K 2001 Violence in mental health care: are there any solutions? Mental Health Practice 5(2):20–22

Howitt D 1998 Crime, the media and the law. John Wiley, Chichester

Independent inquiry into the death of David Bennett 2003 Norfolk, Suffolk and Cambridgeshire Strategic Health Authority, Fulbourn, Cambridge

Laurance J 2003 Pure madness: how fear drives the mental health system. Routledge, London

McIness S 2001 The political is personal: or why have a revolution (from within or without) when you can have soma? Feminist Review 68:160–180

Markham D, Trower P 2003 The effects of the psychiatric label 'borderline personality disorder' on nursing staff's perceptions and causal attributions for challenging behaviours. British Journal of Clinical Psychology 42(3):243–256

Martin J P 1984 Hospitals in trouble. Blackwell, Oxford

May D, Kelly M P 1982 Chancers, pests and poor wee souls: problems of legitimation in psychiatric nursing. Sociology of Health and Illness 4:279–299

Mills S 2003 Michel Foucault. Routledge, London

Morrall P 2000 Madness and murder. Whurr, London

Rowden R 2003 Fears raised over plan to 'dump' women patients at Rampton Hospital. Mental Health Practice 7(4):5

Shifrin T 2005 A need to see the patient rather than their offence. Nursing Times 101(40):46–47

Shoenberg E 1980 Therapeutic communities, the ideas, the real and the possible. In: Jansen E (ed.) The therapeutic community. Croom Helm, London

Strachan-Bennett S 2005 RMNs still await rules on restraint. Nursing Times 101(48):10

Taylor P J, Gunn J 1999 Homicides by people with mental illness: myth and reality. British Journal of Psychiatry 174:9–14

7

Responding to a confused patient: what would Aristotle have done?

Necessity is the mother of invention

(Horman 1519)

PART 1: ARISTOTLE'S ETHICS

Aristotle's preoccupation with the sensible world – what Bryan Magee (2000) called 'his love affair with experience' – reflected his opposition to abstract constructs as not helpful in practical appraisals of everyday moral problems. His ethics invites us to consider how people's day-to-day beliefs impinge on their situations and influence moral choices. For Aristotle: 'It is the way that we behave that makes us just or unjust' (Aristotle 1955, 1103b1–25) and he insists that there is nothing in the intellect that is not first in experience. For example, he stresses the importance of habit formation in how people come to make judgements. It has been said, almost as a truism, that no occupational group is as much a creature of habit as nurses.

Aristotle's great contemporary, Plato, took another view altogether. For Plato, morality lay at the mercy of abstract ideas of what constitutes right and wrong. He postulated an unchanging 'other worldly' realm of Forms (or pure ideas) which have their pale reflections in our world of constantly changing objects. For Plato, it is to these Forms that our reason appeals when we deliberate on life's problems. It is not surprising that it was Platonic ideas which fitted better the formation of Christian doctrines of right and wrong. That said, Plato's ideas could also bring him up short. For instance, he had to contend with the problem of applying abstract principles to practicalities. It is here, when he grapples with issues of intent and culpability – practical applications of law – that he is forced into line with Aristotle's view. Plato held that criminal acts are unintentional – most of us do wrong because we are out of touch with the Form of Knowledge, familiarity with which would enable us to do the right thing. However, he was unable to square this with how the law was applied to intentional as opposed to unintentional acts. So he allows distinctions between these in the sentencing of criminals, a principle that underpins jurisprudence to this day. Perhaps desirous that philosophy not be held up to ridicule (Barker 1960), he allowed that criminal intent ought to warrant greater punishment than crimes perpetrated through passion or ignorance. We shall see (towards the end of this chapter) that claims to ignorance do not justify abusing patients' rights or infringing their wellbeing. But, given that, as psychiatric nurses, we intend to do something, to take some action in respect of patients, it is still worthwhile asking how we know what the right thing is to do. And it is this question of intent, operating within ethically charged settings, which concerns this chapter; specifically, the extent to which a consideration of Aristotle's teaching might aid nurses in their deliberations and help them make right choices.

KNOWING WHAT TO DO

Aristotle believed that an elite of Greek males (of whom he was one) will know what is the right thing to do but he says little about what others must do, or about moral order generally. As Rowe (1991, p. 127) observes: 'Greek ethics is about bridging an individualistic ethos with the demands of the institutions of the city state.' In effect, Aristotelian philosophy hardly concerns itself with morality at all (at least not as we would know it) but, instead, addresses what some (men) must do to attain *eudaimonia*, a word usually translated as 'human flourishing'. In *The Nicomachean Ethics* Aristotle writes: 'We are studying not to know what goodness is, but how to become men' (Aristotle 1955, 1103b26). This is what human flourishing is: across the life-span a state of virtue is attained by which the individual brings his society (the moral order) into alignment with his self-perceived status as a significant figure within that society. The oddness of how this nowadays sounds provoked Bernard Williams (1981) to charge that Greek thought 'lacked the concept of morality altogether', a remark too far, considering that Aristotle's stress on the importance of social factors in attaining 'the good life' suggests *some* concern with a moral order operating outside the agent or at least influenced by the agent. True, his concern is to unravel the nature of the individual's adaptation to society's demands and this is not the same as constructing external rules by which we might live: rather is the intention, always, to ensure that power relationships between individuals and society are weighted unequally towards the individual. This is a philosophy, therefore, that calls for individuals to act from virtue, from a sense of what is or is not the right thing to do. It relies less on abstract systems of ethics such as deontology or utilitarianism, being grounded in the lifelong personal search for a balance between self-goodness and the demands of the world. It is a balance that has to be worked at; at no time is it easy to establish.

DIFFICULTIES WITH ETHICS

Aristotle believed that ethical rules 'hold only for the most part'; he knew that inductive thinking was alive to the possibilities of contextual influence (and events) that might refute whatever generalisations induction pointed to. At first glance, his doctrine of the mean constitutes a yardstick by which choices can be made. This doctrine states that for any given choice there is a middle way but, typically, the virtuous man must find this himself; the mean cannot be established outside individual reasoning. As such, it is not a 'proper' (arithmetic) mean at all since it is rooted in subjectivity. However, 'the continent man abides by his own calculations' (Aristotle 1955, 1145a34) and the mean allows some evaluation of the relative amounts of reason and desire in making decisions. The incontinent man, alternatively, knows when he does wrong. Ignoring the mean (but not ignorant *of* it), he places desire above principle; he does not follow reason. Either way, the situation is fundamentally egotistical, denoting a style of social engagement and very much rooted in its own time. As such, its philosophical usefulness to nursing practice might seem, at first sight, to be limited. This is not so and over the last 20 years or so MacIntyre (1985), among others, has argued that virtue ethics – placing personal virtue at the centre of moral decision making – broadens the scope for arriving at right answers. MacIntyre's *After Virtue: a Study in Moral Theory* (1985) was timely for nurses in that it paralleled significant aspects of nursing's professional evolution. In particular, virtue ethics fitted the kinds of holistic thinking then emerging within nursing, during the 1980s, and its 'new departures' in educational curricula and codes of conduct. For nurses, virtue ethics (i.e. Aristotle) was back in business.

TIME

Although constantly faced with moral dilemmas in their work, psychiatric nurses are often unable to withdraw from the workplace so as to reflect on or analyse the issues. They must make right choices on the basis of available facts and there will be instances where, in the white heat of the moment, reflecting on the basis of abstract systems such as deontology or utilitarianism may simply be impracticable: nurses may, as it were, have to fall back on themselves. For instance, a nurse may have to act to prevent a dementing patient wandering off into danger. In such circumstances, Aristotle would emphasise the dispositional elements of responding. In effect, I prevent the dementing patient from wandering into danger because I am disposed to do this. I have become, through habit, the kind of person that maintains patients' wellbeing. Many nurses lay claim to this kind of moral stance, perhaps calling it something like 'knowledgeable doing'. Reason is necessarily present in these cases since, if I reflect on my actions, their rightness will be confirmed. And even if there is insufficient time to reason, the nurse's disposition to protect their patients (to which we may add some concern about being held to account) will impel them to act in the right way. Some might say that the issue of accountability places the discussion within a consequentialist type of ethics, for example utilitarianism. However, in this case, accountability is not about consequences since the nurse *reasons* that not to take action is wrong in itself even if, in the second instance, it is potentially culpable. Having said that, it is conceded that consequentialism, to some extent, must play its part in *any* ethical choice. To deny this seems psychologically questionable.

IRRESOLVABLE DILEMMAS

If Aristotle believed that ethical issues were grounded in the perplexities of daily living, like other Greek philosophers and many philosophers since, he was reluctant to identify right moral actions, preferring instead to describe procedures – such as his idea of the mean – by which people might choose. Rowe (1991) suggests that it is at this point (of imprecision) that ethics becomes interesting and that Aristotle's 'nothing can be done' position enhances philosophical problems because of the challenge of their irresolution. Aristotle's notion of imperfect moral rules shadows Hursthouse's (1979) concept of irresolvable dilemmas, dilemmas that appear to dissolve when subjected to abstract systems like deontology and utilitarianism. The latter eliminates conflict by converting moral questions to equations such that 'good' equals 'the greatest good of the greatest number'. Deontology, alternatively, suggests that when we take an action we do it in such a way that the act could be applied universally. Both of these systems are more satisfactory to some because they are perceived as rigorous and testable. For example, the deontologist will insist that promise keeping be made universal, that a world in which we could break some promises would make nonsensical the very notion of promise keeping. Utilitarians on the other hand might insist that we have no obligation to keep a promise to a murderer if lying would prevent further destruction.

Although both of these approaches can be vigorously defended, neither seems to capture the complex texture of much moral experience. There is an absolutist quality to both in how they exhort us, respectively, to *always* tell the truth or to *always* side with the greatest number. True, utilitarianism allows us to evade issues that are singularly uncomfortable by adopting the greatest good rule but only at the expense of the residual doubt that we have slid past the problem, avoided its irresoluteness. An adequate ethics should allow for irresolvable dilemmas because this more realistically apprehends questions of choice. People do not emerge unscathed from their moral dilemmas and these can assume tragic proportions if what is to be decided is too terrible to be called right or good and the agent, although having acted well, is left with what Hursthouse calls 'moral remainder'. Deontology and utilitarianism proceed as though people can discard their 'psychological baggage' and think and believe in abstract ways. This is the joke embedded in the characterisation of Mr Spock in the television series *Star Trek*, the fun of watching someone behave without feeling, operating purely on logic. The weave and web of human exchange extends beyond logic, owever. Who, outside of Kant, a major deontologist, thinks as a Kantian, leaving aside all notions of consequences when making moral decisions? And what of the utilitarian deciding that a medical treatment be withheld from a learning disability patient and be given, instead, to someone who isn't and then moving on without any experience of conflict? By conflict I don't mean regret from having had to make a decision but rather the psychological hangover born of the irresoluteness of the actual decision taken and the doubt that one *has* acted rightly.

PART 2: THE DILEMMA

An elderly patient – admitted voluntarily to an acute admissions psychiatric unit – may have progressive Alzheimer's disease but may, alternatively, have a recoverable toxic confusional state. He refuses to go to the bathroom and is, because incontinent, showing signs of tissue damage from urine acidity. All efforts to persuade him to wash have failed. Some of the nurses believe that his tissue damage reveals negligence on their part. In addition to being concerned about how others – relatives, managers – may view this, they believe that leaving the man in this state violates the principle of beneficence, the practice of doing good, acts of charity towards others (Beauchamp & Childress 1994). On the other hand, respecting his decision not to wash contributes to the patient's autonomy. However, concepts of autonomy in any moral definition carry the implication of informed consent. In this instance, while the patient is legally entitled to refuse treatment, his mental status is uncertain: he may have a (recoverable) toxic state; at the same time, he may be in the early stages of dementia. The implication is that if it is the former, then his non-compliance is not completely uninformed given the temporary nature of his mental state. What this issue of temporariness does is force a comparison between the 'here-and-now' – what is happening in the lives of persons now – and who they are across the life-span. Aristotle's principle of 'the good life' invites us to look to the whole life of persons (Aristotle 1955). That is to say, the nurses' actions should not be governed just by who a patient is at a point in time. That, even if demented, *who he has been* contributes (to an extent) to who he is now. In addition, who (or what) he may become also counts when proposing to treat him or give him care. This is not to abandon decision ethics altogether but to suggest that the 'here-and-now' fails to capture the profundity of ethical choices when considering people across the life-span.

DISTRESSING

The patient is confused (for whatever reason) and that confusion will lead to distress if he is forced to bathe. And not only distress for the patient. In a similar case reported by Inglis (2000) a decision to use force incited conflict among the nurses involved. Believing that they had acted with beneficence these nurses also felt that they had violated their patient's autonomy. Although not intending to do wrong, they could not completely escape the thought that they had saddled themselves with 'moral remainder'. Whatever the moral complexities of intention – and they are considerable – psychologically, it is always difficult to be exact about one's intentions without elements of self-deception and doubt creeping in and around one's thoughts. Can these nurses, for instance, be sure that they have ruled out considerations of how their actions – whatever their form – are not, a result of their anxiety at being seen as inefficient? In addition, some psychologists do not separate human cognition from feelings (Forgas 2000) so that reasoning is never completely free from hormonal, nervous system or social mediation. Indeed, is it likely that humans can execute detached, formulaic decisions in response to ethical dilemmas in the way that some philosophers – for example the deontologist Kant – suppose? Plausibly, one can universalise a law about truth telling such that it is always our duty to be honest. There is an abstract clarity to this, however, that seems to vanish when one approaches the practicalities of living. How, for example, does one universalise a rule that all incontinent people of like circumstances be acted upon in the same way?

In the present case, one way to resolve the conflict is to abandon autonomy on the grounds that, because mentally ill, the patient is not acting from reason. This is a familiar psychiatric strategy where the elements which contribute to a (Kantian) good will, in particular the absence of extraneous forces influencing rationality, are held not to apply because of a presumption of psychotic pathology. Yet the patient's confusion – if due to external toxins – is temporary and it is questionable if temporarily confused people forfeit all rights to their views being taken seriously. In my opinion, they possess a residual autonomy based, first, on their retaining *some* capacity to reason (the patient is not speaking gobbledygook, for example) and, second, on grounds of having exercised autonomy in the past as well as perhaps doing so again in the future.

The idea of taking the longer view is linked to Aristotle's insistence that we deliberate on means, not ends, and if we do deliberate on ends we should do so as a means towards further ends; what is needed to achieve an immediate end revolves around the further ends to which satisfaction of the immediate end is aimed. However, this presupposes some underlying agreement about what ultimately the good end is – the final Good – and it poses the question of whether nurses would espouse what is good differently to how others would do this. Some nurses might force a patient to wash not as an end in itself but as a restorative act which ensures that the patient attains a more dignified, psychological and social status. These nurses would utilise force because they care for the patient sufficiently to overcome their anxieties (and his objections) in acting for his ultimate benefit. They would say that they would act this way from an 'ethics of caring', that they are a 'caring profession'. Bradshaw (1996, pp. 11–12) sums this up thus:

> "The … content and direction of care have been our nursing heritage, a foundational assumption, however little articulated; an altruistic compassionate love concerned with the needs not only of the cheerful, helpful, and grateful patient or client, but also of people who may be unattractive, ungrateful, unhygienic, awkward and demanding."

This follows Aristotle inasmuch as the central question is not 'what is the right thing to do?' but 'what will the (virtuous person) do?'. This is because there is no one solution that is right; a range of actions are permissible any of which will be right because carried through from virtue. Recognising that there are no easy answers, the virtuous person inculcates and rehearses the virtues using reason as the final arbiter. In the case of nurses, in addition to reason, some might derive ethical sustenance from feminism or from some religious perspective. For Bradshaw, it is the latter; for Patricia Benner (1984), an influential nurse theorist, it is the former. However, it is difficult to see how these perspectives work in respect of our incontinent patient because it cannot both be right to leave him sitting in urine *and* take him to the bathroom and to then justify either action by protestations of caring whether underpinned by religion or feminism. On that basis, a concept of caring could be used to justify anything. This is unsatisfactory not just because essentially subjective but because it avoids naming objects or ends to which it is subject: it does not say what it cares about.

OBJECTS OF CARING

According to Peter Allmark (1998, p. 13):

> *"Judgements are not made upon the absence or presence of care in itself. A caring person cares for the right things in the right way."*

In other words, an ethics that simply enjoins one to care is devoid of content; carers must state what they care *about* because the object of their care might be objectionable. For Bradshaw (1996) an ethics of caring is bolstered by Christianity and it is true that the Judeo–Christian tradition underscores many ethical systems. But, of course, Christianity doesn't just admonish us to care; it sets out rules which enjoin us to care in particular ways and about particular things. It doesn't operate in an abstract bubble and, unsurprisingly, much of Christian doctrine is underscored by Aristotelian thought.

Emphasising the object of caring challenges the usefulness of virtue ethics in ensuring right actions and there has been something naïve about the uncritical acceptance of caring theories by nurses, the easy assumption that nursing is somehow synonymous with goodness. In fact, assuming the title 'nurse' is no guarantee of virtuous behaviour as we know from the past. For example, the history of psychiatric nursing is littered with physical and psychological abuses of patients in institutional care (Martin 1984, Stanley & Penhale 1999). Some, following Plato, might say that our immoral acts stem from not knowing the right thing to do. This, however, plays down how pleasure can motivate bad behaviour: if we are driven to satisfy desires at the expense of nobler impulses – and it seems that we are – then it looks as if we do need moral yardsticks to control our baser instincts. An ethics of caring, alternatively, bereft of indicative rules or ends, would not take one in one direction or another. If a patient was in pain, a nurse might act to end that pain by administering a lethal injection – because he/she cared. Equally, the nurse might attempt to end the pain but also strive to maintain life – because he/she cared. What this suggests is that ethical codes, whether derived from Christianity, feminism or the Nursing and Midwifery Council (NMC), are not sufficient to deal with moral dilemmas.

A further complication is that while issues of life and death may be relatively clear cut, the dilemma of the incontinent patient is not and it may be that Allmark (1998) supposes that determining the objects of caring is relatively straightforward when, in some cases, it is not. Further, even when claiming an ethics of caring, it is unlikely that anyone acts without considering what *counts* as good or bad. Allmark (1995, p. 13) concedes that we commonly call actions 'caring, careless, uncaring' and it is unlikely that nurses would not be cognisant of some of their actions being seen as immoral despite claiming to 'care'. Where the issue is relatively unambiguous – ending a life – then statements of the kind 'I did it because I cared' are not enough. That said, our courts are normally lenient when euthanasia is seen as an impetus to care by (and for) a relative. In the case of the incontinent patient, I am not sure that nurses *can* know what is the right action to take: compelling arguments could be made for washing him (forcibly) or for leaving him alone.

ROOM FOR MANOEUVRE

Part of the difficulty is that nurses may not have the occupational freedom to determine the sources of their concerns, whether these concerns derive from their knowledge of and relationships with their patients or the need to evaluate how their actions will be seen by others. Determining the scope of nursing, in settings influenced by politically driven treatment outcomes, occupational norms and medical necessity, can be problematic. That nurses *can* exercise objectives, possess the space to determine right courses of action, is uncertain. For example, in psychiatric settings they will be hamstrung by organisational and historically determined demands on their role (Clarke & Flanagan 2003) as well as multiple legal requirements. In the present case (and climate) many nurses would certainly be keeping an eye on the consequences of their actions. Neither the patient's relatives nor hospital managers will take kindly to the patient remaining unwashed. The traditional functions of nurses seem clear and their nervous awareness of the patient's physically deteriorating state will press them into washing him. But what of their moral function, the 'readiness to do fine deeds'? Is leaving this patient to his own devices defensible on the grounds of respecting his autonomy? Or is his (perhaps) temporary confusion sufficient reasons to forcibly wash him? If his medical status is that he has Alzheimer's disease does this make it more likely that force will be used? Perhaps. What if his refusal is due to equal parts confusion *and* cantankerousness? How do you distinguish between the two in terms of what is motivating him to refuse? What *are* the differences between delusion, confusion and straightforward refusal?

KNOWING AND DOING

Knowing that their actions violate his civil liberties means that the nurses must be certain that when they do this it's done from a caring impulse that is directed towards (the objective of) his wellbeing. However, distinguishing certainty from arrogance is difficult and 'caring' may become a euphemism for expediency. Yet doing nothing seems hardly an option: the nurse must act since, in effect, not to act is equally to act and the result may be seen as negligence. Aristotle provides some refuge from this when he says that 'the field of deliberation is what is practicable for the agent, and that the actions are for the sake of something else' (Aristotle 1955, 1112b26). A urine-soaked patient is not practicable in a nursing context but a forced removal constitutes an assault on his autonomy (not to mention his dignity). But there is loss of dignity already, his being incontinent in a public place, and the resultant tension reflects the need to balance the sources of indignity and choose wisely between them. A utilitarian response would nullify this ethical angst and the patient would be washed since why should the unit as a whole have to suffer inconvenience? If this sounds abrasive, the alternative is to act well towards the patient, perhaps not in the instant but with an eye to the long term. Self-cultivating virtue seems to be what Aristotle is about. To be virtuous is to use one's reason; one cannot act ethically simply from an impetus to care. That said, reasoning may not make actions good in clear cut terms; our best hope is to believe that what we do in the here and now – in this case, violating a patient's autonomy – is done with the final good of the patient in mind.

TYPES OF RESPONDING

Moral philosophers typically 'sit on the fence' when it comes to providing solutions to the moral dilemmas they raise: happy to describe types of moral responding, what would satisfy this or that ethical system, but rarely saying what they would do. This, of course, allows them to avoid the charge of professing moral expertise and the pitfalls that doing that would produce. Indeed, when philosophers do throw their ethical 'hats into the ring' they arouse suspicion as much as admiration: witness such examples as, say, Russell, Sartre or Heidegger. While not desiring to, preposterously, put myself in their company, I feel nevertheless that I should say what I would do in the circumstances. In my view, leaving the patient to fester in urine is not an option although I am unable to *argue* why; there is an insoluble quality to the problem in that, whatever one does, there will be much left that will rankle. However, to act against the patient's wishes, provided this follows upon considered reflection by a multidisciplinary team (involving families brings on an entirely new range of problems), will prevent physical and social deterioration and/or distress. But it will be psychologically distressing to the patient nevertheless, damaging to his dignity, and morally ambiguous.

ARISTOTLE AND THE INCONTINENT MAN

Aristotle assumes that we have the power to choose between different courses of action but he alters the rules by which we can know which action to take in different circumstances, for example circumstances where we are relatively free to choose as against choices made under duress. His method is to discuss matters of a general nature but in respect of a particular case. In addition, he rejects the notion that the higher moral good is something that only an elite can possess; rather, the moral 'high ground' is attainable by us all. Therefore, he sees it as perfectly natural that, in working through moral problems, we should rely heavily on experience. This is what moral actions are about: dealing with issues in the here and now, working our way through social encounters and their ethical dimensions.

This is also why it is important to give credence to people's moral views, both as evidence of what needs to be done in a given situation but also as building blocks for constructing a picture of what counts as morally good. It was Plato's view that a small number of men aspire to goodness by acquiring knowledge of the Form of the Good; for Christians this would translate into Commandments handed down 'from above'. Yet, in real terms, this is constantly opposed by the contingencies of the situations where problems occur. For some, 'Thou Shall Not Kill' becomes a principle of the highest order. But how principled is it if by not killing – for instance in a just (Hitlerian) war – a greater evil prevails?

Aristotle's philosophy holds that it is difficult to value people in terms of single events; the incontinent man is therefore seen not just in his present predicament. Equally, nurses have cultivated ways of responding which, at their heart, seek to respect the wholeness of those whom they nurse. As such, their responses stem less from arbitrary judgements and more from moral habit. So that whatever action they take is founded on their commitment to the welfare of patients. Given that something has to be done, but that the pros and cons of this are impenetrable, this 'something has to be done' may be the best we can hope for. But, in the case of the patient, it may be reckoned unsound both philosophically and practically: philosophically, because force violates autonomy; practically, because leaving him be violates a) duty to care and/or b) the welfare of others who must suffer his company. Force will probably be grounded in utilitarianism: being left alone stems from a version of duty to care. I would be reluctant to act from a standpoint of 'I was only doing my duty' since these words must surely count as some of the most terrifying in the language.

We could trust in the virtue of the nurse, trust that his/her station will always lead them to act in good ways. Part of the difficulty is the impossibility of knowing people's character: there are many nurses and how can one know, among them, who is good or bad? However, Aristotle's stress on experience and human complexity does provide for working through what might be right behaviour towards this patient even if arriving at a clear-cut solution is unlikely. But at least the insolubleness of the problem provides a retroactive balm, allowing one to say that given the contradictory, albeit equally appropriate, solutions to the problem I choose this one. It does not get rid of, but may yet lessen, residual guilt.

References

Allmark P 1995 Can there be an ethics of caring? Journal of Medical Ethics 22(1):19–24

Allmark P 1998 Is caring a virtue? Journal of Advanced Nursing 28(3):466–472

Aristotle 1955 The Nicomachean ethics. Penguin edition (edited by Thomson J A K). Penguin, Harmondsworth

Barker E 1960 Greek political thought. Methuen, London

Beauchamp T L, Childress J F 1994 Principles of biomedical ethics, 4th edn. Oxford University Press, New York

Benner P 1984 From novice to expert: excellence and power in clinical nursing practice. Addison-Wesley, Menlo Park, California

Bradshaw A 1996 Yes! There is an ethics of care: an answer for Peter Allmark. Journal of Medical Ethics 22:8–12

Clarke L, Flanagan T 2003 Institutional breakdown. Academic
Publishing Services, Salisbury

Forgas J P 2000 Feeling and thinking: the role of affect in social
cognition. Cambridge University Press, Cambridge

Hursthouse R 1979 On virtue ethics. Oxford University Press, Oxford

Inglis S 2000 Nursing ethics. Mental Health Nursing 20(9):18–20

MacIntyre A 1985 After virtue: a study in moral theory. Duckworth,
London

Magee B 2000 Confessions of a philosopher. Phoenix, London

Martin J P 1984 Hospitals in trouble. Blackwell, Oxford

Rowe C 1991 Ethics in ancient Greece. In: Singer P (ed.) A companion
to ethics. Blackwell, Oxford, pp. 121–132

Stanley N, Penhale B 1999 Institutional abuse: perspectives across the
life course. Routledge, London

Williams B 1981 Moral luck: philosophical papers 1973–1980.
Cambridge University Press, Cambridge

8   Legal mischief

Truth lies at the bottom of a well

(Democritus 460–370 BC)

Like most people, I used to think that government policy was carefully thought through, that the rule of law was fair and that our politicians would inform us about diseased food as effortlessly as they would solicit our votes. Not now. Like many people, I now know that public bodies do not always furnish 'the facts', telling us instead what they want us to hear. Today, we inhabit a 'culture of spin', a political landscape where little is as it seems and where much that seems what it is, is not. It isn't just that we were misled about poisonous beef, but that we were deemed so incapable of understanding events that they needed 'spinning' into something more palatable. The masters of deception are the tabloid newspapers and there are two areas where they display their cruel talents to great effect: one is in matters of race and migration, the other being the 'clear and present danger' of 'mad people loose' in the community.

MEDIA

When the mental health organisation MIND (Baker 2000) surveyed over 500 people with different mental illnesses about their views on press coverage, 73% believed it to be unfair, unbalanced and negative with half of them believing that this negativity was deleterious to their health. Although some media outlets, *The Guardian*, *The Big Issue* and *Eastenders*, were seen as fair and unbiased, the tabloids were seen as obnoxious. As Flory states (1998, p. 4):

> *"Perpetrators of acts of violence are often described as 'schizos', 'nutters', 'psychos', 'fiends', 'monsters' and 'maniacs', particularly in the tabloid press, making a clear link between violence and mental distress."*

Foreland (1998, p. 8) suggests that it is the nature of tabloids to push stories that are frightening, their usual method being to:

"Start with a scary statistic that someone is killed by a mental patient every fortnight. It sounds like confirmation of the psycho-killer myth but it hardly survives scrutiny. Tabloid tales of 'crazed killers' are statistical flam, designed to tap into a deep and ancient fear of the lunatic: mad, bad, and dangerous."

Governments, far from defending the mentally ill, often capitulate to these fears presumably for fear of accusations of 'not doing enough', of not 'taking a tougher stand'. In a letter (BBC News 2005) to Professor Graham Thornicroft, Chairperson of the Government's Advisory Group on Mental Health, the then Secretary of State for Health, Frank Dobson, in response to growing fears about mentally ill people 'in the community', proposed a 'third way' of dealing with this 'failure of community care'. This consisted of balancing, on the one hand, proposals for crisis helplines and teams, more hostel accommodation, extra counselling and support services with, on the other hand, more secure units and assertive outreach teams – 'to keep tabs on people'.

NEW LEGISLATION

In addition, he proposed legislation 'to enable carers and professionals to respond promptly and effectively to the needs of mentally ill people'. He then announced a review of existing legislation stating that 'the changes in practice we are seeking will be backed up by changes in the law'. In the event, what this third way achieved was a deflection of attention away from the custodialism embedded within his, Dobson's, statement. As these proposals gathered momentum they also began to garner critics. Writing in *The Independent on Sunday*, Laurance (2002) saw them as a regression into a custodial and punitive past. While a balanced front had been promised, what had emerged from the government's draft bill was a raft of measures seeking to detain people with personality disorders – *presumed* capable of social disorder – as well as permitting forced treatments in community settings. Unsurprisingly, combinations of media hype, public apprehension and sheer misinformation had resulted in government policy that, in Laurance's (2003) view, reflected 'a culture of containment' with rising drug prescriptions, increased detention and custodialism: in effect, a service driven by fear.

The Mental Health Bill was announced in the Queen's Speech in April 2005 despite having being criticised, when in draft form, by a parliamentary committee which warned that it would diminish civil liberties. Yet, although 69 charities, campaign groups and professional bodies petitioned the government (Batty 2005) the bill went ahead. Heralded as an advance in the treatment of mentally ill people, some of its provisions may indeed fulfil this promise. However, close examination of the government's explanatory notes (DoH 2004) reveals a less than enlightened picture. For example, one proposal calls for the provision of a 'nominated person' to speak for named patients. The patient has a fairly free hand in choosing who this will be but to the question, 'should the nominated person have the power to discharge a patient from the formal powers of the bill?' the answer is no. The nominated person may make appeals, formally and informally, but that is that: they will have little power outside that of 'interested party'. We shall examine the apparent downfall of this legislation later. For now, what matters is how mental health law is driven not just by informed opinion and health-care research but by the media's cynical concerns about 'public safety' and the need to 'do more'.

MENTAL HEALTH

Bell (2003) divides media content into two kinds: 'them' stories and 'us' stories. In 'us' stories, he says, we are presented with events that happen to 'ordinary people', events that a presumed audience will identify with. 'Them' stories, alternatively, address that which is assumed to preclude the interests of 'ordinary' people: asylum seekers, for example, will cost 'us' money or they will mug 'us' on the way home from 'our' honest day's toil. Mentally ill people fall into the 'them' category, the underlying assumption being that mental illness belongs to others: we may feel sorry for 'the mad' but remain susceptible to being 'tabloided' into anger and/or fear (*Daily Mail* 2005, *Daily Mirror* 2005) particularly when trip words like 'loonies', 'maniacs', 'psychos', 'fiends' are displayed. An especially distasteful aspect of this is their doubling up of effort where the mentally ill offender is male, muscular and black.

Of course, little of this is new; for instance, politicians have always presented things in ways that reflect favourably on them. What has changed is the sophistication of the delivery, the speed at which information is disseminated, as well as the growing scope for public and private institutions to manipulate data to their own ends. Nowadays most aspects of our lives are subjected to advertising pressures: even manufacturers who successfully induced us to smoke stubbornly resisted attempts to curb their hard sell. In the case of governments, spinning material into acceptability has reached the mesmerising heights of wizardry. It ultimately fails, though, because actual agendas, despite the spinning, must eventually come into public view somewhere, sometime. You would suppose that politicians, eager for their place in history, would abandon 'spin' – and, indeed, the present government says it's done this. The belief that this is possible is a delusion, however, because it presupposes a world that is not driven by vested interests of finance and power strategies per se. The point being that 'spin doctors' are but the visible ends of an economic/sociopolitical complex that will always ensure its own survival and prosperity. In other words, 'spin doctoring' is but the system's failure to conceal its mendacities.

Notwithstanding this politics of disenchantment, even cynicism, it was a surprise to discover that the number of killings by mentally disordered people has differed little to what it was 20 or so years ago (Appleby 1999, Taylor & Gunn 1999) and that, indeed, 'lower' homicide rates had been known for some time (Howitt 1998) but had been camouflaged by a media intent on contriving a negative imagery of mentally ill people in the community, fuelling imaginary high numbers of non-existent attacks and killings. The closure of mental hospitals brought an exodus of patients into the community and these have now merged with a second generation (of patients) who, never having seen the inside of a mental hospital, are also trying to come to terms with community life. Although the story of hospital closures has been chronicled elsewhere (Barham 1992) several aspects require further configuration. The move to the community was a troubled transition not least because it re-invigorated ages-old prejudices. While not ignoring the difficulties faced by discharged patients, a number of them, unable to cope with their illness and, now, social exclusion and degradation, took their difficulties out on others. Previously, mental hospitals had absorbed those for whom society had little or nothing to offer. No longer absorbent, and with many community psychiatric nurses case-loading non-psychotic patients, the community became an empty space for those who might otherwise have been segregated. Today, we confront the fall-out from these changes, especially the lack of community resources. The tabloid perspective has made 'the community' a byword for every imaginable fantasy: a place of murder and unease, of loss of control, humiliation, vagrancy and dispossession. Renewed concerns about dangerousness on our streets have provoked responses composed of more compulsory admissions, at-risk registers, increased forensic services and community custodial treatment.

MEDIA CONCERNS

Matters may be improving (the government's proposed mental health legislation has now been abandoned (BMJ 2006) in favour of re-jigging existing legislation and there is also in the media itself a growing concern about black and ethnic minority issues). However, these concerns vary from newspaper to newspaper as well as being generally reactive. At one point, the tabloids highlighted every transgression by mentally ill people and even some by people deemed to be mentally ill. Their inclination is to define aggression as characteristic of schizophrenia and not explicable, for instance, by environmental pressures. Philo (2004), reporting on surveys conducted by the Glasgow University Media Group, showed that associating schizophrenia with violence was traceable to media accounts and that government policies were implicated in these. Although governments have not been party to deliberate scaremongering, be it on ethnic or other grounds, they seem loath to condemn such activity forcefully while seemingly collaborating with them via draconian legislation and a kind of inverse spinning wherein positive aspects of mental illness are left unstated.

Reid-Galloway (2002) adds that when this association is joined by race, it provokes 'extremely negative connotations in the public imagination'. She noted that the tabloids matched words and pictures differently in terms of whether those involved were white or black. Referring to the study 'Care in crisis as mental patients are freed to kill', she noted that the photographs of white perpetrators were often juxtaposed with words such as 'graduate' and 'released' but that pictures of black faces were linked to words such as 'violent' and 'stabbing' and she concludes (p. 1):

> *"The stereotype of the 'big, black and dangerous' man is not new, but it has recently been powerfully reshaped into the image of the man who is 'big, black, mad and dangerous', an image that has part of a strong racist undercurrent in public debates on mental health."*

Laurance (2003) names the Christopher Clunis case as a watershed whose impact led to major attitudinal changes among mental health providers as well as the general public. In 1992, Clunis, just released from hospital detention, killed a man on the London underground. His case was seen as seminal in bringing concepts of dangerousness and risk to the forefront of political and professional debate. However, disturbingly, Clunis, a large black male, had his face continuously emblazoned across every tabloid. In a comprehensive analysis of British newspapers Edward Maliki (1992) demonstrated how the tabloids had become keen to publicise violence by young black males, stigmatising this group as uncontrolled, malevolent and threatening. The manner by which Clunis was portrayed came shamefully close to suggesting that blackness was the embodiment of madness (Neal 1998). Neal's paper also locates prejudice within wider historical constructs, arguing that prejudice is a carry-over from imperialist notions of white superiority and the inferior status of black and conquered peoples. The civilising mission of imperialism was to assess and categorise colonials and 'colonial psychiatry' played its part. Fanon (1986) argued that colonialism of itself breeds pathology but it had no shortage of help from psychiatrists who looked to the 'African mind' as prone to madness and incapable of self-government (Chaiklin 1997), who diagnosed such things as 'frontal lobe idleness' and, in the Americas, Cartwright's infamous drapetomania (Cartwright 1851). Not for nothing were psychiatrists originally called alienists or that multiple descriptions abound for the mentally ill as not being of this world. This sense of alienation and otherness is deepened when as an outcome of prejudice the individual concerned can be *seen* as not one of us.

AMBIVALENCE

More recently, press concerns might more accurately be described as ambivalent. For example, it's not uncommon for newspapers to challenge racial stereotypes while simultaneously aggravating white anxieties that reinforce those stereotypes anyway:

> *"It is in and through representations, for example, that media audiences are variously invited to construct a sense of who 'we' are in relation to who 'we' are not ... By such means, the social interests mobilised across society are marked out from each other, differentiated and often rendered vulnerable to discrimination."*

(Neal 2003, p. 59)

In other words, preoccupation with race is frequently aligned with mental health and especially with real and imagined incidences of violence and aggression. That said, these associations are on the wane and race – although not violence – is beginning to lose its vibrancy. Johanna Clarke (2004) recounts the case of boxer Frank Bruno initially labelled 'bonkers Bruno' by *The Sun* newspaper (*The Sun* 2003, p. 1) only for the paper to change its tune following protests from mental health pressure groups. No doubt, 'loveable' Frank's fame and popularity played against racist depictions. Yet *The Sun's* positive response to criticism – whether from genuine concerns about racism and mental illness or from anxiety lest its circulation fall – still reflected a shift in attitude. And when, in May 2005, Glaister Earl Butler, a black male convicted of killing a police officer, was detained indefinitely, *The Sun's* reaction was muted. Putting the story on pages eight and nine, the paper nevertheless couldn't contain its liking for emotive language: its headline ran 'Five mistakes that let psycho kill a cop' (Parker 2005). The *Daily Star* equally removed the story from its front page to page eight but with the headline 'The blunder that left knife fiend free to butcher a cop' (Lawton 2005). The *Daily Mirror* was equally informative: 'Violent, paranoid, scared, dangerous: why was he freed to murder a copper?' (Chaytor 2005).

AGGRESSION

Of course, for those directly affected by violence perpetrated by mentally ill people, the consequences are truly tragic. But as victims' relatives sometimes point out, the answer is not to blame individual patients; rather is it about looking at how and why the community has failed to accommodate their needs adequately and how this can be improved. The National Schizophrenia Foundation (2005), for example, points to shortages of community accommodation, lack of employment and poor crisis management, arguing that these require urgent attention. If these are the real factors implicated in patients' distress, then proposals to treat people involuntarily are an avoidance of the more socially complex work that needs to be done.

While standards of community care have been discussed ad nauseam, the question of who, in psychiatric contexts, is or is not fit to live freely in society has not. Historically, the asylum/hospital was both a custodial and therapeutic place where mentally ill or socially unproductive people could be accommodated and treated. Hospitalisation at least plausibly diminished questions of patients' civil rights since it could be assumed that those treated involuntarily were *unable* to function in society: legislation provided for their detention and treatment because they were a danger to themselves or others. It is asking a lot of psychiatric nurses that they impose compulsory treatments in contexts where patients are deemed fit to live in society. It is especially worrying that they be required to use force in order to implement physical treatments. According to (then) Home Office Minister, Paul Boateng, current legislation does not 'entail, in practice, distressed patients being held down against their will and forcibly injected over their own kitchen tables'. However, there is much still in the government's proposals that is sowing seeds of confusion and repression: witness, for example, the assertion that 'a modern legal framework must offer the flexibility to tackle unacceptable risk to personal or public safety wherever it occurs', or Mr. Boateng's claim that 'the law must make it clear that non-compliance with treatment programmes is not an option'. Mr Boateng was noted by the *BMJ* (Warden 1998, p. 365) as saying:

"We must make sure we do not allow a culture of non-compliance ... which precipitates breakdown. If you [patients] are to remain in the community ... you must complete your medication ... If you don't the law must give clinicians the power to bring you back into a place of greater safety for yourself and the wider community."

Putting some of these proposals (not all) on the back burner, as the government has done, in no way implies their abandonment and indeed it has been announced that proposals will be interwoven into existing mental health legislation. According to Professor Nigel Eastman of St George's Hospital, London:

"The government's climb down on reform of mental health legislation is, almost certainly, merely a prelude to climbing up by another route."

(*BMJ* 2006, p. 737)

In particular, the government may resist pressures to include in the amended law principles of autonomy and reciprocal rights so as to enhance the ethical standing of the legislation. Professor Eastman urges us to remain vigilant, to scrutinise in great detail the provisions of whatever is proposed. He concludes:

"There is a grave danger of being lulled into a false sense of security through having apparently won the seven year phoney war. The real parliamentary battle is about to begin."

(*BMJ* 2006, p. 738)

AND AFTER THE VIOLENT ACT, WHAT?

For many, compulsion will amount to no more than persuasion. However, inasmuch as compulsory community treatment means physical treatment, and allowing that some patients will refuse absolutely, then physical force will sometimes be required. That being the case, the prospect of nurses entering someone's home and forcibly 'treating' them, the police cuffing them prior to their being injected and in a context where they continue living at home (and what that implies) is morally dubious. And after the violent act, what? How to respond when the patient says 'shame'? We are, after all, talking about free people here, people who may happen not to want treatment, whose intransigence, such as it is, is not necessarily symptomatic of illness.

To be free is to be able to choose: community treatment orders say 'you are semi-free, fit to live freely but not quite, not without medication'. In effect, the provisions of the asylum/hospital become a community-wide therapeutic bureaucracy, a virtual asylum whose boundaries are fixed as effectively by statute and, ultimately, custom and practice as by bricks or mortar.

IN SUPPORT

Compulsion, of course, has its supporters. Peter Morrall (1998) argues that psychiatric nursing has persistently disowned its historical task of 'policing the mad' and he has a point. However, his analysis ignores undercurrents of resistance to custodialism, for example those nurses committed to the therapeutic community ethic. My own research (Clarke 1996) into forensic nursing revealed prodigious conflict between those relishing their custodial obligations as against those who sought an ambiance of counselling and psychological support. The latter reflected the training and interests of the younger nurses, true, but also their nervousness about how custodialism affronted professional standing and therapeutic embarrassment.

THE NEGLECTED PRAGMATICS OF ENFORCEMENT

A lack of pragmatism attends discussions about community-enforced treatments. Most, for example, assume a fairly compliant patient; however, outside hospital contexts, a patient's resistance is psychologically different for two reasons. Firstly, the hospital was there to be got out of; therefore, cooperation brought its rewards and compliance had its advantages. The community is an open 'system' and so compulsion requires permanent surveillance. The hospital, its bricks and mortar, was an easy focus for debates on its inadequacies whereas, disseminated throughout the anonymity of community, repressive instincts are more rather than less likely to flourish since they are more diffuse and less permeable to critique and review.

DUTY TO CARE

Because it becomes difficult to sustain beliefs about dangerousness and its outcomes many will fall back on beliefs about 'duty to care'.

A particular danger of this 'duty' is that it can justify treating anybody, from the dying to the unhygienic, and it actually takes little account of what patients want. Its beauty, of course, is that it can be utilised in support of patients who do not want treatment at all, the duty to care benevolently invalidating their view as a lack of insight. Few can deny the appropriateness of community supervision for patients who are a danger to themselves or others. However, current proposals for compulsory treatments rest on assumptions that patients *may* become dangerous to self or others. But can it be right that patients who stop taking medication be coerced into changing their minds because professionals *anticipate* deterioration if they don't? If so, doesn't this signal the end of therapeutic relationships where the decisions of all involved are respected? It is said that imposing treatments will occur only rarely and as a last resort. However, as Tony Heath (1998) says, that it will occur at all goes some way towards defining what psychiatric nursing is. And again, if it is going to be such a rare event, why the need to enshrine it in law? Either I'm missing something or we're not being told the full story.

References

Appleby L 1999 Safer services: national inquiry into suicide and homicide by people with mental illness. Department of Health, London

Baker S 2000 Environmentally friendly. MIND, London

Barham P 1992 Closing the asylum: the mental health patient in modern society. Penguin, Harmondsworth

Batty D 2005 Controversial mental health reforms back on the agenda. The Guardian, Tuesday May 17th, p. 8

BBC News 2005 Online. Available: http://news.bbc.co.uk/1/health/141651.stm

Bell A 2003 Us and them. British Medical Journal 326:291

BMJ 2006 Editorial: Reforming mental health law in England and Wales. British Medical Journal 332:737–738

Cartwright S A 1851 Report on the diseases and physical peculiarities of the Negro race. The New Orleans Medical and Surgical Journal (May), pp. 691–715

Chaiklin H 1997 Colonial psychiatry and the African mind. Journal of Nervous and Mental Disease 185(8):528–529

Chaytor R 2005 Violent, paranoid, scared, dangerous: why was he freed to murder a copper? Daily Mirror, May 20th, p. 11

Clarke J 2004 Mad, bad and dangerous: the media and mental illness. Mental Health Practice 7(10):16–19

Clarke L 1996 Participant observation in a secure unit: care, conflict and control. Nursing Times Research 1(6):431–440

Daily Mail 2005 Maniac freed to kill. Daily Mail, February 26th, p. 1

Daily Mirror 2005 Freed for an hour to kill. Daily Mirror, February 26th, p. 17

Department of Health 2004 Draft Mental Health Bill: explanatory notes. Cm6304, Department of Health, London

Fanon F 1986 Black skin, white masks. Pluto, London

Flory L 1998 Public attitudes to mental distress. MIND, London

Foreland J 1998 Out of the bin and glad to be mad. The Guardian, January 21st, p. 8

Heath T 1998 Compelling arguments. Mental Health Care 2(1):10–11

Howitt D 1998 Crime, the media and the law. John Wiley, Chichester

Laurance J 2002 Mental health: the fear factory. The Independent on Sunday, June 30th, p. 4

Laurance J 2003 Pure madness: how fear drives the mental health system. Routledge, London

Lawton G 2005 The blunder that left knife fiend free to butcher a cop. Daily Star, May 20th, p. 8

Maliki E 1992 Content analysis of British newspapers: ethnicity and mental health. Annual Conference on Mental Health. English National Board for Nursing and Midwifery. York St. John's College, Ripon

Morrall P 1998 Mental health nursing and social control. Whurr, London

National Schizophrenia Foundation 2005 Lost and found: voices from the forgotten generation. National Schizophrenia Foundation, London

Neal S 1998 Embodying black madness, embodying white femininity: populist (re)presentations and public policy – the case of Christopher Clunis and Jayne Zito. Sociological Research Online 3(4). Online. Available: http://www.socresonline.org.uk/3/4/2.html

Neal S 2003 The Scarman report, the MacPherson report and the media: how newspapers respond to race-centred social policy interventions. Journal of Social Policy 32(1):55–74

Parker A 2005 Five mistakes that let psycho kill a cop. The Sun, May 20th, pp. 8–9

Philo G 2004 Changing images of mental distress. Glasgow University Media Unit, University of Glasgow, Glasgow

Reid-Galloway C 2002 The African Caribbean community and mental health in Britain. MIND, London

Taylor P J, Gunn J 1999 Homicides by people with mental illness: myth and reality. British Journal of Psychiatry 174:9–14

The Sun 2003 Bonkers Bruno locked up. The Sun, September 23rd, p. 1

Warden J 1998 Mental health law to be tightened. British Medical Journal 317:365

Ethnicity, race and the paddies

9

Diaspora: a way of thinking about mental distress in migrants

'Tis distance lends enchantment to the view
and robes the mountain in its azure hue

(Campbell 1799)

DIASPORA: DEFINING THE TERM

Diaspora is a concept of migration and resettlement that seeks not just to map migrational movements of people but to also understand their social deprivation, human sexuality and psychological experiences. My underlying assumption is that without appreciating people's hinterland, the myths and imaginings they carry from their pasts, obtaining a fuller understanding of their psychic distress will prove difficult.

Diaspora means dispersion and is applied to populations whose social, economic and political networks cross nations, even span the globe. Fundamentally, the concept transcends the nation state as the primary unit of analysis of migrants, their movements and cultural evolvement. Classically, it accounts for the language and the history of Judaism. As Baumann (1997, p. 377) puts it:

> *"The term Diaspora interprets not only the land, across which one is dispersed, but also the activity of dispersion as well as the people, who are dispersed ... put in a nutshell, diaspora constitutes a Jewish theology of exile."*

However, this usage has expanded in recent years and, outside its Jewish roots, obtains wider currency around the 1960s when it examines the origins of black slavery. Eventually, the criteria of

Diaspora widened to include factors such as involuntary exile to two or more foreign regions, an experience of loss, the development of collective myths about homeland and an ongoing yearning to 'go back'. The experience of loss is important because, although not all migrations are involuntary, attention has tended to focus on so-called 'victim Diasporas': Jews, Africans, Irish.

DISPLACEMENT

Geographical displacement leads to a search for unblemished, idealised images of pre-displacement life. But rather than reclaim identities grounded in reality, to the extent that this is possible, Diasporic groups tend to form constructs that enhance communal self-esteem and self-worth: 'the past' dignifies the group as it searches for its displacement status (Davis 2004, pp. 185–186, pp. 194–195). For example, through contemporary art forms such as music, Afro-Caribbeans forge identities ingrained in their pasts but which also merge into larger, host cultures. Appiah (1992), for instance, argues that there is no pure African culture any more than that there exists an American culture without African roots; from this perspective, confrontational contrasts between a unitary Africa and a monolithic West are misguided as are assertions of *pure* dissimilarity between Irish and English populations. Diasporic thinking, therefore, focuses on identities grounded in dissonances through which migrant and host cultures continuously produce and reproduce themselves to each other; this is particularly true for the young whose desire to absorb host cultures while retaining transgenerational influences is problematic. Such difficulties were well captured in the movie *East is East* (Ayub Khan-Din 1999) where pasts and presents both conflict and connect across cultural and racial barriers. For Professor Stuart Hall (Davis 2004) forging identities in this way is real; people, he says, *can* change and he points to alterations in Caribbean consciousness from the 1970s before which he had (p. 186):

> *"never once heard a single person refer to themselves or to others as, in some way, or as having been at some time in the past, African."*

To which may be added, for our purposes, the acquisition of Britishness as an expansion and contraction of Afro-Caribbean history and culture; in effect, the construction of a social matrix whereby cultural distinctions are both diminished and enhanced.

ETHNIC FORMS

Thus does a Diasporic approach shoot holes through racial specificity by positing hybridist cultures that dispense with national boundaries. In a sense, the Diaspora becomes a method for investigating links between identity and place; it shelters the subgroup's dynamic while allowing it to work through its relationship to the host environment. It allows one to manoeuvre between (and against) two understandings of pedigree: for example, identifiable elements of black music are not only transported across nation states but are transformed and made responsive to indigenous forces.

It's a perspective that has not gone unchallenged. For example, many black-techno musicians are critical of white European and (even) Detroit performers whom they accuse of making 'soulless, simplistic, imitations of techno'. Gillen goes further, asserting that techno 'has so much black culture in it that you can't say it could have happened anywhere else' (Tausig 2003, p. 5). What is being said here is that white appropriation of black music rejects black consciousness as incapable of encompassing white experience; as such, Eminem's rap is what Hooks calls 'white cultural imperialist appropriation of black culture' (Childs & Williams 1997, p. 80). This particular debate, among others, reflects the tensions which inform Diasporic relationships, tensions which betray struggles between ascendancy and oppression, between hybridity and separateness.

RECAPTURING THE EMERALD ISLE

A particular tension is the juxtaposition of negativity and self-inflatedness that occurs within Diasporic groups. The Irish in Britain, for example, live in the heartlands of the perceived oppressor; at the same time, they entertain remembrances of things past, of belonging to an Irish 'land of Saints and Scholars'. They experience the fallout of second-class citizenship (Bracken & O'Sullivan 2001, Greenslade 1992) whilst being cognisant of a homeland 'tiger economy' that boxes 'above its economic weight' in both Europe and the world. It is a paradox fuelled by loss and hope: there is a feeling of belonging to the host country – perhaps signified by material possessions or social role – but in the sense of what Vertovec (1999) calls 'decentred attachment'.

Fintan O'Toole (1997, p. 130) describes an Irish exhibition in New York where soil from 'the old country' is on display:

> *"In a room in a city in another continent, there is still an overpowering sense of Ireland. The very stuff of the land has*

become, not less but more tangible, not more abstract but more real. The soil trodden on heedlessly so many millions of times, the earth that was scraped off boots or washed off potatoes, has acquired the awesome magic of authenticity."

And it is the connection with *there* which fuels the sense of what it means to be *here*. It is where the Diaspora learns to speak to the host culture, to articulate a politics of plurality: a plurality, however, which insists that the problematic origins of migration be camouflaged; thus, the myth-making and idealisation of homeland which confers on the subculture its sense of presence, however hangdog this might be.

GENDERED EXPERIENCES

Few empirical studies address the nature of mental distress amongst Irish communities in Britain. Those that do normally emphasise clinical perspectives and diagnosable illnesses. More rarely (Mac an Ghaill 1996, Williams 1996, Williams & Mac an Ghaill 1998), attempts are made to represent Irish communities across indices of occupation, class, gender and risk, relating these to broader concepts of psycho-social distress. For example, taking the second wave of Irish immigrants into Britain (during the 1950s and 1960s) we can see that males quickly became identified as low-class manual workers whereas, fairly quickly, women ascended the social ladder through middle-class endeavours like clerical work, nursing and teaching. According to Mac an Ghaill (1996, p. 47) 'workplaces are the crucibles in which male identities take on shape and develop meaning'. For Irish working-class men, identity took hold within occupational slums whose surface, visible, conditions exacerbated notions of 'Paddy' as feckless, dishevelled, un-bright, and dangerous. For these men, work meant the construction industry and, because subcontracted as labourers, they lacked the security of occupational permanency as well as being exposed to health risks (including death) through accidents (DoH 1993). Some dealt with this by exaggerating maleness in terms of physical strength, a 'boys sticking together' rhetoric, seeking solidarity in masculinised units such as pubs and clubs with their rebel songs and mixtures of hardman/sentimentalism fuelled by alcohol.

GAY ALIENATION

It was within this context that Mac an Ghaill (1999) examined a cohort of 30 Irish migrant gay men in their twenties living in

London. The study is notable for the light it casts on cross-cultural exchanges including issues of sexuality, occupation, class and identity. Employed mainly within service sectors, these gay men were unable to lock into the more typical representations of Irish male gendering. Indeed, their misgivings amounted to an aversion to Irishness with its disproportionate stress on masculinity and aggressive resistance. Rather did they feel more comfortable inside the London gay scene even when that scene sometimes rejected them for their Irishness. Interestingly, such rejections and accessions also proceeded along class lines, with working-class gay men less able than their middle-class colleagues to blend into the gay scene. For the middle-class group, entrée to the scene was made easier by an ability (and willingness) to pattern new identities, their 'belongingness' now attached to issues of consumerism, interpersonal and intrapersonal styles of language, fashion and ethics. In effect, Diasporic processes were pushing them towards a composite identity possessed of existing as well as acquired strands of culture. Yet this does not obliterate the predicament of those unable to get the balance 'right' and, even now, thousands of Irish migrants remain homeless, on the streets, and/or in need of psychological support (Bracken & O'Sullivan 2001). Yet a concept of Diaspora at least fosters a dialectics by which these issues are now publicised and attended to, as well as providing Irish groups with a method, and the confidence, to articulate their position. What we need now is a shift from middle class, articulate groups experiencing social or sexual exclusion to those relegated to psychiatric categories of psychosis, alcoholism and so on. The issue is urgent because the Irish community have the highest rates of mental illness for all ethnic groups in Britain. Because multicultural policy in Britain has 'embedded visible difference as the salient marker of ethnic difference' (Howard 2006) little attempt is made to capture and define the mental problems of a white Irish community within a socio-political Diasporic milieu or to ameliorate the gross social problems which stem from clinical approaches that ignore ethnic status.

All of this applies equally to those now collectivised as 'asylum seekers' as they too struggle for social adjustment and acceptance. It must be tempting for them to 'circle the wagons' and denote their culture in exclusive terms. God knows, given the ethnic abuse they face, you could hardly blame them. However, a concept of Diaspora, of reciprocity between host and migrant groups, may shrink some of the tensions of migrant status and allow for explorations of (and possible solutions to) the higher than usual incidences of socio-mental distress that cruelly attend that status.

References

Appiah K A 1992 In my father's house: Africa in the philosophy of culture. Methuen, London

Ayub Khan-Din 1999 East is east. Miramax Films, London

Baumann M 1997 Shangri-La in exile: portraying Tibetan Diaspora studies and reconsidering Diaspora. Diaspora 6(3):377–404

Bracken P J, O'Sullivan P 2001 The invisibility of Irish migrants in British health research. Irish Studies Review 9(1):41–51

Childs P, Williams P 1997 An introduction to post-colonial theory. Prentice Hall, London

Davis H 2004 Understanding Stuart Hall. Sage, London

Department of Health 1993 The health of the nation: accidents. HMSO, London

Greenslade L 1992 White skin, white masks: mental illness and the Irish in Britain. In: O'Sullivan P (ed.) The Irish world wide: history, heritage, identity. Vol. 2. Leicester University Press, London, pp. 201–225

Howard K 2006 Constructing the Irish in Britain: ethnic recognition and the 2001 UK censuses. Ethnic and Racial Studies 29(1):104–123

Mac an Ghaill M 1996 Irish masculinities and sexualities in England. In: Adkins L, Merchant V (eds) Sexualising the social: power and the organization of sexuality. Macmillan, London, pp. 122–144

Mac an Ghaill M 1999 What about the lads? Emigrants, immigrants, ethnics and transnationals in late 1990s Diaspora. Paper given at Emerging Irish Identities Conference. Trinity College, Dublin

O'Toole F 1997 The exile of Erin: images of a global Ireland. New Island Books, Dublin

Tausig B 2003 Detroit techno: race, agency and electronic music. Online. Available: http://www.umich.edu/~historyj/pages_folder/F2003_issue.html

Vertovec S 1999 Three meanings of 'Diaspora', exemplified among South Asian religions. Diaspora 6(3):277–300

Williams L 1996 The economic needs of the Irish community in Birmingham. City Council, Birmingham

Williams L, Mac an Ghaill M 1998 Health accommodation and social care needs of older Irish men in Birmingham. The Irish Government's DION Fund and Focus Housing Group, Birmingham

10 Constructing mental illness in Irish people: race, culture and retreat

Happy is the country which has no history

(Benjamin Franklin 1740)

THE APPEAL TO MADNESS

In the past, Irish people used mental hospitals more frequently than their British counterparts. Whether this indicates an increased prevalence of mental illness or a peculiarly Irish 'appeal to madness' is an issue whose solution is fraught with difficulty. The fact is, many reasons have been advanced to explain the almost symbiotic relationship between madness, the Irish and mental hospital admission rates. In John Millington Synge's *The Playboy of the Western World* (1981), for example, the appeal to madness becomes a 'solution' to social, and particularly familial, problems, it being assumed by the play's characters that the main character's physical attack on his father must be the work of a 'madman'. But more so is their lionisation of Christy and his probable patricide symptomatic of an unconscious 'yearning' to escape drudgery and boredom, to use Christy as a totem for wishful thinking and projection. Mercier (1962), in *The Irish Comic Tradition*, declares a comic intellectual heritage through Swift to Shaw, Wilde, Joyce, O'Casey, Flann O'Brian, Beckett and Heaney: comic spirits unfazed by ambiguity, psychological dislocation or even death. Kearney (1985) asks whether history imposes this or if it is a quality of Irish thinking. Something of both, I suspect, although the received wisdom today is that the qualities of ethnicity are culturally determined and change as history unfolds.

By the end of the 19th century, Irish mental hospitals were chock-full of inmates and the phenomenon was not lost on western observers and investigators. For example, in his analysis of the Omagh Lunatic Asylum for 1895–1905, Prior (1996) found that its inmates were predominantly small Catholic farmers and unskilled labourers, mostly bachelor males within the age group 20 to 50. In terms of the aetiology and diagnosis of these patients matters remain vague but most of them showed patterns of disruptive family relationships that are faintly reminiscent of the types of psychosis described by R. D. Laing (1960) in the 1960s.

POST FAMINE

The story of mental hospitals in Ireland must be set against the post-famine changes occurring after the 1850s. Finnane (1981, 1996), for instance, notes that large-scale post-famine emigration, and consequent rural depopulation, reduced the capacity of families and communities to care for their mentally unwell. Thus, the county asylum may have provided a temporary refuge or retreat for those who otherwise would have famished.

This element of retreat is important. Many Irish people (even today) go on religious retreat; such retreats are seen as a means of replenishing the soul (and the psyche). It is conceivable that these religious 'outings' siphoned off a psychological distress that might otherwise have propelled some towards psychiatric care; equally, it is feasible that behaviour normally construed as psychotic might have been protected through parochial perspectives of what is merely odd or eccentric. This leads towards a folkloric concept of people's oddities and fripperies, radically misperceived and enshrined in anthropological studies and the emergence of so-called 'west of Ireland schizophrenia'. We will see (Ch. 11) how conventional psychiatry responded effectively to this phenomenon using point prevalence methodology and careful comparisons of samples. However, there exists a rich anthropological tradition which takes its lead not from quantifiable approaches but from social constructionist and other socio-cultural perspectives: in essence, approaches which regard mental illness as constructed from family and/or wider social dysfunction. For example, one approach has analysed correlations between 'schizophrenia' and the non-married state in males (Murphy & Vega 1982), inferring that patterns of marital/sexual dysfunction lead ultimately to pathological beliefs which resemble schizophrenia. Almost all of this social research has been carried out in rural Ireland, with urban centres generally avoided.

DECLINE OF RURAL COMMUNITIES

Commins (1986) urged caution when differentiating between urban and rural since social class, and their economic correlates, might be determinants of behaviour irrespective of rural or urban living. However, size characterises what counts as 'rural' (usually less than 1500 inhabitants within a given area) and so it is hard to ignore isolation in how one construes change. The extremes of isolation are most noticeable in the west of Ireland where as many as three quarters of the people live rurally albeit against a background of constant migration to urban centres. From the 1940s these communities became a focal point for western, particularly American, anthropologists eager to expose their internal dynamics and perceived conflicts. Among the most celebrated of these was Nancy Scheper-Hughes' (1979) study of a small isolated village in Co. Kerry. Using Durkheim's concept of anomie (1989) Scheper-Hughes (1979) set out to describe excessive rates of schizophrenia in this community. The village she chose, having assessed the suitability of several, was a tightly knit and socially aware village but which possessed the quality of being cut off, nestling, as it does, at the edge of the Atlantic Ocean on the Dingle peninsula.

Scheper-Hughes' descriptions of its people are especially poignant in respect of young and middle-aged bachelor farmers. These small farmers are commonly bolstered by government subsidy with many of them on welfare. A consequence of Ireland's entry into the European Economic Community (EEC) is that many of them would face early retirement; they would receive the market price for their farms which would then be amalgamated into larger collectives, leaving the smallholders adrift, displaced, dispossessed.

Reminiscing on the death of his home town, Charlestown, Healy (1988, p. 71) recorded the following exchange between two of its villagers:

> 'I hear the Land Commission finally got Charlie Henry's place.'
> 'Aye. Sure it must be an ease to poor Charlie – what was in it for him on that holding? He's better off in England.'

Healy notes that Charlie's farm was an uneconomic proposition at the best of times and, at worst, but 'one small corner of a decayed rural slum which now makes up the hinterland of Charlestown'. An added worry is that there never was in Ireland a concept of retired farmer: elderly folk would continue to make their presence felt in the running of their own or their offspring's farms. Indeed, inactivity was equated with immorality and retirement looked on as moral death. Long life was ascribed to hard work and Scheper-Hughes recorded villagers' legendary stories of dying men deciding to have a last look at, for instance, a new-born calf only to discover that once 'on their feet' they became, once more, 'right as rain'. This 'rebirthing' is hilariously dramatised in John Ford's classic film *The Quiet Man* (1952) where an old-timer lies dying. About to expire, he hears the distant roar of a fist fight between the film's two main protagonists; with acrobatic abandon, he charges from his deathbed, trousers half on, half off, gleefully re-invigorated, once more ready for the fray.

SOCIAL ANOMIE

The deterioration in rural life and culture has been interpreted as a 'decline in rural fundamentalism' (Commins 1986). It was a fundamentalism that comprised positive views of:

1. the family-run farm as the basic unit of agricultural production
2. large numbers of farmers
3. farming as an occupation
4. agriculture as the basis of national prosperity
5. farm or, at least, small community living.

These were the principles that inexorably surrendered to industrial economic planning as well as to cosmopolitan perceptions of agricultural life as 'backward'. So that it wasn't just science and technology, prices, incomes and industrialism that negatively impacted on rural growth and diversity but, as well, modernist values which increasingly defined Ireland in urban terms. Industrialisation accelerated secularisation as well as preoccupations with materialist explanations of what does or doesn't work. The role of religion (and mystery) in people's lives diminished and with it the place of myth, but especially the home-to-home gatherings that made the reshaping of myth, through story telling, an important means of social cohesion.

Of course, these changes were hardly unique to Ireland: from Donegal to Africa industrialisation and wealth production effectively cut the village:

"*off from its roots in the traditional agrarian society of the past.*"

(Buruma & Margalit 2004, p. 112)

What has not been recorded is the extent to which these processes were validated by the long line of studies which reified these communities as odd and psychologically discordant in terms of western Euro-American norms.

THE STUDIES

Arensberg & Kimball (1940) set the tone by describing Irish communities as integral forms, their internal social alignments and inclusiveness complete almost as if pre-ordained. It was a perspective bordering on the pastoral: an Ireland quaint and cosy, warm and simple, dependent on work, barter, religion and 'sports'. But we can doubt the extent to which these 'ordered societies' reflected underlying realities, whether in fact they reflected the fictional projections of researchers in search of a Celtic Shangri-La. Reviewing John Ford's film, *The Quiet Man* (1952), Henry Hart wrote that:

> *"Ford reveals ... a way of life, stable, rooted, honourable, purposeful in nature's way, and thereby rhythmic. Everyone is an individual, yet everyone and everything has a place."*

> (Haliwell 1995, p. 829)

The film is less idyllic than this: it is suffused with sexual, religious and ethnic tensions sometimes only barely concealed. But this is denied by those who seek more stereotypical notions, who prefer superficial readings which fit more easily the happier regions of the imagination. The community of one's heritage is an imagined place which can telescope smoothly into the realities of the present. A community's history, wrapped in story and song, contains enough self-fulfilment to induce conformity with imagined characteristics of the past. Thus the suspicion that Irish/American anthropologists were insufficiently rigorous, rendering descriptions that confirmed predetermined views.

Yet, at face value, there was probably much that seemed to them quaint and out of step with their experiences of normative social progress. One factor that invariably caught their eye was 'the arranged marriage' and, branching out from it, communities sustained by mutual aid and reciprocal generosity. Researchers were inclined to interpret interruptions to these 'undisturbed' patterns as destructive; occasionally, as in Ford's film, the initial disruption is caused by an outsider, in this instance the son of emigrants who returns home. (Upon his return the entire film then turns on his relationship with a squire's sister and his failure to understand local permutations of courtship and marriage.) Sometimes matters are less clear.

Brody (1973) describes a 'demoralisation' that resonates inwardness, an inherent melancholy, not something external or superimposed. At the same time, the effect of political/economic change, the growing amalgamation, mechanisation and commercialisation of farms, makes its presence felt incrementally. Since society can no longer supply their wants or needs, so have people lost the need to be bound by its norms. Having lost faith in the continuance of social order, they withdraw from it; with anomie (Durkheim 1989) there is a failure to understand the meaning of things. Brody shows this failure occurring not by exclusion as much as through realising that one's place has ceased to have meaning. Of course, Brody too may be a victim of beliefs about organic completeness and its disruption by modernisation. But while allowing for some exaggeration, there did prevail a 'peasant model' of farm life, its main features being:

1. a family economy (i.e. not employing labour)
2. subsistence (not commercial) production
3. arrangements for the transfer/inheritance of property
4. locally bound mutually supportive relationships between neighbours.

Whatever the full 'facts' of farm life, this list reflects a norm of sorts. The problem is that 'gilding the lily' assertions about rural interdependency play down its harsher, meaner, subsistence elements, the kind of picture that comes from Patrick Kavanagh's (1972) poetry where the one constant is graft, scrimping and scraping for a meagre living, nothing idyllic at all, only bleakness. (Kavanagh, incidentally, hated Synge's 'idyllic' portraits of rural life, which he considered unrealistic.)

A PEASANT CLASS

Until the 1960s, it was a failure of economic expansion which provoked rural decline. When small farms failed there was little their inhabitants could do but leave. However, it is not just a material equation: there was also a psychological incapacity to understand and deal with decline apart from drifting into alienation and withdrawal (O'Connor & Daly 1983). For example, impoverishment made arranged marriages more difficult, although such marriages were on the wane anyway, increasingly rejected by a growing, post-peasant, female emancipation. The result was a forced flight of the young, especially young women, to England and whereas, in the past, they might have returned with a marriage dowry, by the 1940s, and certainly the 1950s, there was little likelihood of their returning at all.

In Brody's (1973, p. 93) study, girls 'openly and remorselessly' reject the marriage offers of local farmers, choosing migration to the city instead. Brody reported not a single marriage for the community he studied for the only time in 150 years. Commins (1986) reports that during the 1950s, rural depopulation was heavy with many areas losing as much as 60% of their young people. Scheper-Hughes (1979) found, in one parish, a total of 64 bachelors over 35 years old with 27 unmarried women in the same age bracket (nine spinsters and 18 widows). Moreover, where she noted over 30 eligible men between 21 and 35 there were only five unattached women between these years with none of them willing to take a local man. Hence, the propensity to depart for pastures new.

SEXUALITY

Women in these communities were often repelled by the shyness and sexual ineptitude of the village's young men, whose awkwardness in their presence could be startling. The Catholic Church had set an age for the attainment of reason (i.e. the capacity to sin) at seven years and with particular emphasis on sins of the flesh – and not just actual sins either. One could sin by entering an 'occasion of sin'; that is to say, one was culpable by placing oneself in a place or context wherein sinning was more likely. With fatalism like this, small wonder that one went ahead and sinned anyway. But it was a dangerous game to play since the punishment was said to be deadly and *forever*: thus was one marked with a central message of the damned, delivered with such force (and repetitiveness) that it stayed with you forever. It helped foster in Ireland what Larkin (1972) has called a 'devotional revolution', one outcome of which was that, by the 1930s, over half of all men and three quarters of women born at the turn of the century were single. While the evidence for 'devotional revolutions' is impressionistic the population of mental hospitals at the time reflected these single/marital statistics; further, it was a phenomenon that persisted. Scheper-Hughes (1979) observed that the most remarkable feature of mental hospitals was the celibacy of their inmates and she cited the 1971 Irish National Hospital Census figures of 88% and 80% single status for men and women respectively. Whatever about revolutions, it is undeniable that religious orthodoxy powerfully affected people's lives both in private as well as publicly. For example, stringent censorship governed many recreational pursuits from public (theatre, cinema) to private (novels, newspapers). School teaching played its part in religious indoctrination with little interference from parents – what interference there was (usually protests about excessive corporal punishment) was resented. Parental affection was hardly absent but was invariably undemonstrative. In his play, *Philadelphia Here I Come!*, Brian Friel (1967) portraits a son about to leave for America at a time when such leavings were seen as permanent. Friel shows that what passes between father and son does so without much being said. Kevin O'Nolan (1973, p. 31) captures something of this in a short biography of his brother Brian (a.k.a. Flann O'Brian):

> *"Our mother died in 1956. I remember Brian asking helplessly how we ——-s deserved or came to have the mother we had. There was no answer. He thought for a long time of writing something about her but it baffled him. Some things are beyond words."*

Irish people of a certain generation (or perhaps temperament) will recognise the non-expressiveness, bottling up affection, things best left unsaid, if not unfelt.

MELANCHOLY

Omnipresent in Irish anthropological studies is dejection: like a wet dog unable to shake itself dry, moroseness sits on people's backs like a hump. So do the middle-aged bachelors in Scheper-Hughes' study indulge in an alcoholic melange of self-pitying recrimination, petitions directed to the past, to what might have been: 'if only' and 'if it wasn't for' digressions which only deepen the mire of their depression. Hugh Brody (1973, pp. 32–33) depicts this:

> *"A drunken man ... leans more heavily on the bar. He often seeks to draw another drinker or two to his side. Such a group creates a tight circle of privacy around itself – a privacy physically expressed by the arms they lay across one another's shoulders. Then, with faces almost touching, they appear to join closely in evident despair. This despair is not expressed in discussion ... rather they exchange silence as if it were words."*

One is tempted to believe that this picture is fast fading, that anthropological sleuths would be hard put to find it now. However:

> *"Today you can see them still, propping up the bars in village pubs, these 'mountainy men' in their later years, often leading very isolated lives, many clinically depressed, suffering from 'the nerves' as it is called ..."*

(Ardagh 1995, pp. 109–110)

The reference to 'later years' is telling though and descriptions like these are becoming unrecognisable as the years wander by. The importance of this 'Celtic melancholia', however, is the extent to which it was seen as a precursor of mental illness, even psychosis.

This, however, is the nub of the matter: it had never seemed (to me) to be clear if, in these studies, we are confronted with psychosis as much as with behaviours endemic to isolated and customised communities, behaviours which had, until the coming of western psychiatry, persisted as peculiarities of habit.

Visiting Ireland with her son, novelist Edna O'Brien (1978, p. 24) came across a:

> "... Roscommon man in a deserted pub ... a madman by his own definition who had lodged there for years ... 'Take that nice smile off your face,' he said to my son and was of a mind to clout him for being so affable. He said, and his eyes were darting, that we were 'snottynoses' but that he knew the subject, predicate and object of any sentence. The other lodger who had been there for ten or fifteen years was gone with his nerves. This is Godot land."

The origins of such 'madness' are never clear although mythical tales of 'being away with the fairies' or being possessed by a 'blessed sickness' held sway for generations, providing explanatory yard-sticks for those willing to believe them or unable to believe anything else. What the visiting sociologists brought to this was a barrage of psychosocial concepts duly applied – with confident brushstrokes. Whether they found insanity or eccentricity, who knows? They did unearth psychological factors, set against a harsh agrarian terrain, that *seem* to bring about mental distress. In his poem *The Great Hunger* (1972, pp. 34–35) Patrick Kavanagh portraits attachment to mother, furtive sexuality and the drudgery of labour:

> "O he loved his mother
> Above all others.
> O he loved his ploughs
> And he loved his cows
> And his happiest dream
> Was to clean his arse
> With perennial grass
> On the bank of some
> summer stream;
> To smoke his pipe
> In a sheltered gripe
> In the middle of July—
> His face in a mist

> *And two stones in his fist*
> *And an impotent worm on his thigh.*
> *But his passion became a plague*
> *For he grew feeble bringing the vague*
> *Women of his mind to lust nearness,*
> *Once a week at least flesh must make an appearance.*
> *So Maguire got tired*
> *Of the no-target gun fired*
> *And returned to his headland of carrots and cabbage*
> *To the fields once again*
> *Where eunuchs can be men*
> *And life is more lousy than savage."*

In Scheper-Hughes' (1979) study, the men are cold, reserved and behave 'oddly' in the presence of women; on social occasions such as dances, the men and women separate for conversation and, for the men, excessive drinking. Catholic asceticism may not have helped here; preoccupation with sexual purity precluded intimacy: these dances were, after all, occasions of sin. We may observe how traditional Irish dancing is asexual, the arms rigidly held at the sides, the dancers barely touching. Organised dances at the time would have been chaperoned but, of course, probably increasing the fun of transgression when and wherever it occurred. Gradually, traditional dancing would disappear, although waves of 'dirty dancing' hardly followed in its wake. For years afterwards, large, well-lit ballrooms became the venues for 'showband' dances with 'jiving' a suitable substitute for the 'hands by the side' method.

MARRIAGE

Marriage, anywhere, is a complex business; research into Irish rural life found it doubly so. First was the unmarried, celibate state and its implications for mental health. Second, marriage was complicated by existing kinships and their connection to land, inheritance and ownership. Casting a family net over strangers was problematic; if marriage was in the offing, and the prospective wife brought to the male's household, such a 'stranger' could be rejected in favour of the blood family. Some were sibling farms with the sister a kind of domestic manager for her worker-brothers. When Scheper-Hughes asked one woman with four brothers why she had never married, she replied: 'What! exchange four healthy men for just one?' So:

1. no marriages
2. no children

3. natural attrition through death
4. migration of the young

led to rural enclaves largely composed of bachelor farmers. This is the group with the highest loading for anomie, at highest risk of psychological distress. Scheper-Hughes (1979) describes a shame, guilt-ridden socialisation which entraps some of these men into staying on their farms. It is a socialisation that defends the mental health of girls and first-born males, the latter the favoured 'white-haired boys' as opposed to the last born, or 'leftover sons'. Scapegoating reduces the status of the leftover son to one who is loved but seen as generally incompetent. The ineptness becomes ingrained, forcing him to turn inwards, his 'headland of cabbage' becoming his comfort zone. In due course he will come to care for his parents, locking into their needs and demands: in effect, he embarks on a second childhood. Travelling through Ireland in the 1950s, novelist Heinrich Boll came upon one such man. Observing him, Boll (1983, pp. 35–36) wrote:

> *"From far off, when he comes in from the meadow with the cattle, he looks like a youth of sixteen; when he turns the corner and enters the village street you feel he must be in his mid-thirties; and when he finally passes the house and grins shyly in at the window, you see that he is fifty."*

Having learned that this man has only a limited awareness of life outside his farm, Boll continues (p. 36):

> *"He goes off again, a man of 50, transformed at the corner into a man of 30, up there on the slope where he strokes the donkey in passing he turns into a youth of 16, and as he stops for a moment at the fuchsia hedge, for that moment before he disappears behind the hedge, he looks like the boy he once was."*

'Double bind theory' (Bateson et al 1956) explains some of this. The mother tells the child that he is loved but discourages affectionate responses; touching is especially discouraged. Conflicted by contradictory messages, the child displays ambivalence or withdraws into make-believe 'where eunuchs can be men' and where he acquires some control. According to Laing (1960), this proceeds to an existential insecurity of such penetration it induces psychosis.

> *"Called to his face a wretched, unfortunate ungainly soul, a leftover, miserable remnant of flesh, the 'old cow's calf', is caught in a classical double-bind in which he is damned if he does and damned if he does not. The parent can be observed*

belittling the runt for trying to put himself ahead and then with the same breath chiding him for not being more aggressive and achievement-oriented like his older brothers."

(Scheper-Hughes 1979, pp. 184–185)

If the runt leaves home, he is the guiltier for having abandoned his parents yet if he stays, he ensnares himself within a consensus of failure to establish his independence. Of course, it is possible to reinterpret this as a style of perpetual sulking: self-pity mitigating responsibility for alcoholism, unemployment, sexual destitution and isolation. The Irish are said to be good at blame; it is *always* someone else's fault.

THE NATURE OF SCHIZOPHRENIA

The nature of schizophrenia can be discussed in medical (Crow 1980) and cultural (Foucault 1971) terms. Many today assert a genetic influence in its development and see the issues as working out the degree of genetic loading with some scope left for social and psychological factors. Scheper-Hughes, however, was committed to an integrative/psychoanalytic approach and she believed that the origins of the disorder lay within family relationships, themselves skewed by wider cultural/religious/economic stresses. This was hardly new, of course; Laing & Esterson's *Sanity, Madness and the Family* (1964) had supplied a powerful rhetoric of family conflict underpinning acute madness states. More empirically, Leff (1976) had documented the effects of family pressures on schizophrenics arguing that, whatever the genetics involved, an understanding of the historical life of the affected individual was essential to any understanding of the disorder. However, the potential for getting it wrong is increased when that 'understanding' fails to extend itself beyond theoretical constructs developed in isolation from the societal mores and historical antecedents of those being researched. In this sense, Ireland can be added to the list of those cultures pregnant with 'exotic salience', almost an invitation to discover the inexplicable, the picaresque, enchantment, mysteriousness.

IN DUBLIN'S FAIR CITY

It's said that when Americans fly into Dublin Airport their ongoing journey through the city centre constitutes a rude awakening. For in that short journey, the savage apparition of spreading industrialisation assassinates their romanticist longings for green grass and greener values. Such things must wait until they reach the tourist heartlands of west and south Ireland where expectations of 'the ould sod' variety will be assuaged by knowing combinations of naïvety and cynicism.

Among the Irish, preoccupation with yesteryear can vary from a 'South Dublin' cosmopolitan view of the past as priest-ridden, superstitious and base ignorant, what John Waters (1991) calls 'a bad dream, a mild irritation on the periphery of consciousness, a darkness on the edge of town' while, for others, modernity represents the death of basic values, loss of purposefulness and a nostalgia for a more temperate culture. Some farmers, especially older ones, might still wish to work their farms within the old familial model. However, the extended family and communal networks to support such models are gone. Symbolic attachment to land can still outstrip utilitarian value (see Jim Sheriden's film *The Field* (1990) for a depiction of the evocative power of land and its meaning in history and family) but contemporary proposals for rural revitalisation are mere wishful thinking. As Roy Foster (1989) notes, by 1971 30% of the working population was still engaged in agriculture but the rate was declining steeply. Most people now lived in urban areas where, following bouts of 'economic expansion', a landscape surprisingly similar to other European capitals has emerged. It differs, however, in that successive Irish governments have been disinclined to oppose property development and what remains of Georgian Dublin is the bit the commercialists left alone. You do not have to look to Africa or Asia to witness the more brazen excesses of globalisation: just stroll down the most commercialised thoroughfare in Europe, O'Connell Street.

COMELY MAIDENS

It wasn't meant to be that way. In an (in)famous radio speech, Eamon DeValera, a founder of the modern state, spoke (much to the merriment of certain classes today – and perhaps even then) of 'comely maidens dancing at the crossroads' and such like. His would be a Gaelic-speaking people, Catholic, culturally independent, and probably economically backward:

> *"His vision of Ireland, repeated in numerous formulations, was of small agricultural units, each self sufficiently supporting a frugal family; industrious, Gaelicist and anti-materialist. His ideal ... was built on the basis of a fundamentally dignified and ancient peasant way of life."*

(Foster 1989, p. 538)

This was never going to be, of course: even 20 years after DeValera's 1946 speech only 5% of farm dwellings had an indoor lavatory and 80% had no facilities at all. However, the 'Celtic Tiger', a massive growth in wealth and spending power, roared into existence from the late 1980s. Arguments persist about the reasons for this 'success' but few deny that influxes of foreign capital aided by lax environmental controls played their part. Corporate taxes were slashed so as to outbid European 'partners' and, as Foster puts it, 'foreign capital [was] attracted with a vengeance'. But it did end emigration at least and the country started to enjoy itself for once, slurping at the trough of western consumerism and privilege. The downsides are the attendant problems that come with this territory: drug use is rampant in urban areas; family breakdown – facilitated by some of the worst urban slums in Europe – has led to high incidences of crime; and levels of alcoholism continue to rise. It's a world that the anthropologists would hardly recognise, a world in which their characterisations of the Irish as a rustic, homely people, battling against the terrors of modernisation and driven mad in doing so, would be seen today as a social libel.

In 2003, the organisation 'Schizophrenia Ireland' (with the Irish Psychiatric Association) published *Towards Recovery*, a landmark report which suggested that things were moving beyond preoccupations with the meaning and prevalence of mental illness to a position of deciding how best to help people with distress while protecting civil rights. As in Britain, the inclusion of service users has changed unalterably the terrain of what is required even if, as in Britain, matters are still too heavily concentrated in the hands of professionals. In an Irish perspective, these changes have yet to touch the lives of emigrants, many of whom still bear the consequences of their migration in respect of their mental health. To them we now turn.

References

Ardagh J 1995 Ireland and the Irish: portrait of a changing society. Penguin, Harmondsworth

Arensberg G, Kimball S 1940 Family and community in Ireland. Harvard University Press, Massachusetts

Bateson G, Jackson D D, Haley J et al 1956 Toward a theory of schizophrenia. Behavioural Science 1:251–264

Boll H 1983 Irish journal: a traveller's portrait of Ireland. Secker & Warburg, London

Brody H 1973 Inishkillane. Penguin, London

Buruma I, Margalit A 2004 Occidentalism. Atlantic, London

Commins P 1986 Rural social change. In: Clancy P, Drudy S, Lynch K et al (eds) Ireland: a sociological profile. Dublin Institute of Public

Administration in association with the Sociological Association of Ireland, pp. 47–69

Crow T J 1980 Molecular pathology of schizophrenia: more than one diseases process? British Medical Journal 280:66–68

Durkheim E 1989 Suicide: a study in sociology. Routledge, London

Finnane M 1981 Insanity and the insane in post-famine Ireland. Croom Helm, London

Finnane M 1996 Law and the social uses of the asylum in nineteenth-century Ireland. In: Tomlinson D, Carrier J (eds) Asylum in the community. Routledge, London, pp. 91–110

Ford J 1952 The quiet man. Republic Pictures, California

Foster R F 1989 Modern Ireland 1600–1972. Penguin, Harmondsworth

Foucault M 1971 Madness and civilization: a history of insanity in an age of reason. Tavistock, London

Friel B 1967 Philadelphia here I come! Faber, London

Haliwell L 1995 Haliwell's film guide. Harper/Collins, London

Healy J 1988 No one shouted stop! The House of Healy, Achill

Kavanagh P 1972 Collected poems. Martin Brian & O'Keefe, London

Kearney R 1985 The Irish mind: exploring intellectual traditions. Wolfhound Press, Dublin

Laing R D 1960 The divided self. Penguin, Harmondsworth

Laing R D, Esterson A 1964 Sanity, madness and the family. Penguin, Harmondsworth

Larkin E 1972 The devotional revolution in Ireland 1850–1975. American Historical Review 77:625–652

Leff J 1976 Schizophrenia and sensitivity to the family environment. Schizophrenia Bulletin 2:566–574

Mercier V 1962 The Irish comic tradition. Clarendon Press, London

Murphy H B M, Vega G 1982 Schizophrenia and religious affiliation in Northern Ireland. Psychological Medicine 12:595–605

O'Brien E 1978 Mother Ireland. Penguin, Harmondsworth

O'Connor J, Daly M 1983 The West Limerick study. Social Research Centre, Limerick

O'Nolan K 1973 The first furlongs. In: O'Keefe T (ed.) Myles: portraits of Brian O'Nolan. Martin Brian & O'Keefe, London, pp. 13–31

Prior L 1996 The appeal to madness in Ireland. In: Tomlinson D, Carrier J (eds) Asylum in the community. Routledge, London, pp. 67–90

Scheper-Hughes N 1979 Saints, scholars, and schizophrenics. University of California Press, London

Schizophrenia Ireland/Irish Psychiatric Association 2003 Towards recovery. Schizophrenia Ireland, Dublin

Sheriden J 1990 The field. Granada Films, London

Synge J M 1981 J. M. Synge: the complete plays. Methuen, London

Waters J 1991 Jiving at the crossroads. The Blackstaff Press, Belfast

11

Curiosity, fact and myth: the Irish in Britain today

Hope deferred makes the heart sick

(Wyclif 1395)

Although Irish immigrants in Britain present with severe mental health and social problems, both in terms of prevalence and the nature of their difficulties (Doolin 1994), you could be forgiven for not thinking so, given the paucity of information about them and their neglect by all but a handful of transcultural psychiatrists, usually themselves Irish or Irish connected (MacGiollabhDin 1995). For instance, Suman Fernando's (1991) standard text *Mental Health, Race and Culture* gives but a passing glance at Irish immigrants and Littlewood & Lipsedge's (1982) classic text contains but a few references.

Described by the Policies Studies Institute (1997) as 'the most detailed examination of the health of Britain's ethnic minorities available' and by Davey Smith (1997) as 'the most comprehensive study of ethnicity and health yet conducted in Britain', James Nazroo's *The Health of Britain's Ethnic Minorities* (1997) presents no data whatever on the Irish in Britain.

In a major text on nursing and ethnicity (Gerrish et al 1996) Irish people are subsumed under the category 'white' as indeed they are by the Nursing and Midwifery Council. In another nursing paper, Cowley & Simmons (1992) go further and make an explicit separation of ethnic and white populations. In a small but important study Murphy & Macleod Clark (1993) found that many nurses lacked understanding of the ethnic dimensions of their clients' illnesses and that some carried negative views about ethnic minorities. In 2000, Unison called for a 'chief nurse for ethnic affairs' but, again, the emphasis was on black and Asian peoples (Nursing Times 2000). All told, 'agencies in Britain concerned with issues of ethnicity and discrimination have persistently ignored the existence of the Irish people' (Tilki 1998, p. 125).

GOVERNMENTS

Governments have fared no better. The *Patient's Charter* (DoH 1996) called for a recognition of cultural differences among patients, which is fine but hardly a substitute for programmes to deal with the problems involved. In the case of Irish people, *Health of the Nation: Accidents* (DoH 1993a) makes no recommendations even though occupational accidents are listed as unacceptably high for this group (p. 86). In *Health of the Nation: Ethnicity and Health* (DoH 1993b) Irish people are not even mentioned. As Tilki (1998, p. 148) states:

> *"Until official discourses recognise the invisible Irish, the citizens rights to which they are entitled will continue to be eroded and their contribution to the society in which they live will not be in balance with what they deserve."*

Other reports are equally vague. *Working Together* (DoH 1998) announced an 'action programme on racial harassment' and in *Patient and Public Involvement in the New NHS* (NHS Executive 1999) there are recommendations for the working conditions of black and other ethnic groups. But in both of these reports Irish people are either consigned to the category 'other' or simply ignored. They are not identified as a group with defined needs and ambitions.

Most psychiatric interest tends to be directed towards black people, be they Caribbean or African, and Asians, whether British or from elsewhere. So it is ironic that whereas British-born black people are often seen as immigrants (most racists regard place of birth as irrelevant) Irish people receive scant attention from mental health researchers although the Irish *are* immigrants and can present with problems as challenging as any other group. A further irony, of course, is that a lot of Irish would blanch at the very *idea* of being called an 'ethnic minority'.

SKIN COLOUR AND ETHNICITY

In a British context, the Irish differ from other ethnic groups along several fronts; crucially of course, they are white. Ostensibly, being white might seem a step up in the race assimilation stakes. However, skin colour only partially mitigates the superiority of one group over the other largely because differences are grounded in prejudicial propositions about characterological 'deficits', for instance intellectual deficiency: more inferior because more than skin deep, so to speak.

There is a need, as Sashidharan & Commander (1998, p. 285) state:

"to desegregate the terms race, ethnicity and culture, which until now have been viewed as synonymous within health care and social sciences."

In emphasising ethnicity, however, one draws attention from the racial discrimination which black and Asian people face. Historically, Marxism defined ethnicity in terms of colour, with whites set in dominant opposition to black. This meant that cultural differences within white groups were minimised. Yet cultural identity, irrespective of colour, may also determine the occurrence of, and responses to, ill health. True, for black and Asian groups there occurs not only a (self) construction of what constitutes difference but differences are also *imposed* on them. However, to confine studies to black and Asian people leads to them being seen as 'problem groups'. Because, throughout this century, sociologists have emphasised Afro-Caribbean and Asian groups, they have created a tradition of 'over-racialising' research while denying the possibility of white groups being seen as racial minorities. This 'deracialising' of the white race leads to what Mac an Ghaill (2000) calls 'the construction of a narrative of homogeneity on the basis of whiteness'. This problematises matters for the (white) Irish in ways that are radically different from black experience. Since the 1960s, that experience has become more realised as a *black* – that is, not African or Caribbean or Afro-American – experience. This diminishes the essentialism of placing white (European) against the 'otherness' of Africa or Asia and in favour of a more heterogeneous distribution (see Ch. 10). In keeping with this, between 1991 and 2001 ethnicity questions changed in the census so as to reflect varied ancestry, it also, of course, introduced breakdowns of the white population to include Irish. For the Irish, nevertheless, relocation and consequent identity are rendered opaque by skin colour: their white skin makes it easier for them to assimilate and 'go native'.

DISCRIMINATION AND ILL HEALTH

And yet, the Commission for Racial Equality (1997) has reported:

"Since the Commission for Racial Equality was established in 1977, Irish people have been coming to it with complaints of

unlawful racial discrimination. Academic research and official statistics have revealed inequalities in Irish people's experience of the labour and housing markets, the health service and the benefits system. Many Irish people in Britain have also objected to being made the butt of humour and remarks which they find offensive."

Whether versed in ethnic or racial terms, the case for some redress of these issues seems clear.

In general, the physical and mental health of Irish people is poor compared to the indigenous population and most other immigrant groups. On average, a male Irish immigrant to England will die ten years younger than his compatriot who stays at home (Marmot et al 1984). The Office of Population Censuses and Surveys (OPCS 1991) stated that mortality rates for Irish males and females aged between 20–69 were among the highest in Britain. More than a quarter of households headed by an Irish-born person contained someone suffering from an incapacitating illness (OPCS 1991, Owen 1995). Summarising the many hypotheses which surround these rates, Kelleher & Hillier (1996) note the tendency for Irish people to consult their GPs less than the general population. In addition, lifestyles are implicated, Balarajan & Yuen (1986) reporting heavy smoking and drinking rates for men and heavy smoking rates in women; accidents derived from the large numbers working in the construction industry are also high. Owen (1995) points to the higher age rates for post-1950 Irish immigrants and the undoubted correlation between age and some illnesses. However, Owen's analysis of the 1991 OPCS data – when adjusted for age – still confirms the high illness rates for immigrant Irish people. Nothing is certain here but if statistics are even approximately correct, then Irish people emigrate so as to die prematurely.

WHITE MASK

Lee et al (1998) point out that ethnicity is a social construction, its significance determined by the more powerful elements in the society where it arises. As such, it is not ethnicity which determines health inequality but the social and health inadequacies which rise from the classification. Liam Greenslade's (1992) reading of Franz Fanon is that by whatever means colonised people cope with feelings of inferiority, it becomes insurmountably difficult for them to do so as emigrants and particularly where they emigrate to the country of their perceived oppressors. Although Fanon's arguments stem from considerations of black slavery, his description of self-deprecation and worthlessness equally applies to the Irish immigrant experience. And, as we shall see, degrading the Irish – to a subhuman plateau – was a necessary prelude to the manner by which their 'sufferings' (famine, poverty, death of the language) were consistently belittled, in literature, history and sociology.

Immigrant status *confirms* worthlessness, provoking the terror which (threatened) loss of identity brings. If immigrant status is experienced as failure then it is at least plausible that it may proceed to depression. One mustn't generalise excessively because many Irish immigrants carry little such baggage. However, high levels of physical and psychological distress are well established (Cochran & Bal 1987, Finnane 1996) albeit, as stated, hidden and/or denied. This is partly because Irish people don't wish to see themselves as an 'ethnic minority': Owen (1995) reports that, notwithstanding a 'Campaign for Irish Inclusion' in the 1991 Census, only a tiny minority used the 'other' box, most Irish preferring to list themselves as 'white'.

SKIN COLOUR

Of course, skin colour is important here and, generally, indigenous groups are more viscerally comfortable with people who look like themselves while harbouring doubts (and fantasies) about those who don't. In transcultural psychiatric research, some foreign cultures are seen as possessing 'exotic salience' whereby their lifestyles are seen as more interesting, more suggestive of psychosocial uniqueness. Such ideas stem from that global anthropology by which obscure groups living dreadful lives in South American mud huts are made idyllic by anthropological 'workers in the field' who would probably shudder at the idea of western people having to live that way. There's a chapter in Kingsley Amis' memoirs (1991) which rails against the type of travelogue, the 'traveller from afar', who, humble in the face of primitive lifestyles, 'the good life' in situ as it were – eulogises all sorts of inhumanities and bestialities on grounds that because they are alien (to us), they are not subject to our ethics or social standards. Of course, we are all subject to the same ethics: special rates do not apply because you are foreign, black, Protestant or obscure. Actually, one can see excessive interest in black or 'third world' countries as essentially patronising; certainly, one's own group, or groups akin to one's own – Irish, Poles or Austrians – are neglected in the process.

THE IRISH

In the case of the Irish, there are other reasons for this neglect: the Irish have been, one way or another, a millstone around British necks for a millennium and continue to be so. There exists a repulsion/fascination about a group who have frequently brought trouble in their wake. The fascination is palpable; witness the prevalence of 'Irish pubs' and the success of television programmes such as 'Ballykissangel'. Yet, there is ambivalence too; attachments tend to be nervous, tetchy, imbued with something of the quality of 'best leave well enough alone'. Fanon (1986) identifies this wariness as stemming from malevolent misunderstandings rooted within colonial experiences and this idea can also be extended to show how depression is partially mediated through socio-economic factors.

IRISH IMMIGRANTS

The Irish constitute quite a presence in Britain. Estimates of up to 30% have been given for the number of actual English with Celtic blood; other estimates are lower but seldom under 10%. For immigrants, numbers vary but some estimate the number in, for instance, the Borough of Brent to be about 9%: that's a lot. Contrary to what one might suppose, they have little representation within political or other power structures. Indeed, Richard Butler (1994), an Irish psychiatric service user living in Brent, paints a drab picture of neglect, particularly for those with mental health problems. The Irish government seems disinclined to help, and Butler complains that his letters to the Irish embassy go unanswered. Now there are many reasons for this, not the least of which is embarrassment: Butler, after all, is a psychiatric user raising issues – mental illness, stigma and homelessness – which may not be to the taste of first-generation Irish born in England (with their English accents) and who may see such things as a threat to their collective identity. It is easy to forget in a materialist and consumer-driven culture what our antecedents have been. Few remember that 80% of Irish children born between 1931 and 1941 *had* to emigrate. They left to the unremitting relief of governments who could continue to ignore the problems that forced them out (Bolger 2005) and who, indeed, could insist that there were no problems. Only today are these people – perhaps in a context of asylum and European Diaspora – being written back into history in a serious way. Writing in *The Irish Times*, Dermot Bolger (2005) recorded the caution of immigrants, their refusal to speak, as well as the fear of foreigners coming to know the Irish experience as the migrant squalor it really was, and he notes how infrequently this story made its way into literature. Some narratives of this experience are provided, for example, by Catherine Dunne in her 2003 anthology *An Unconsidered People*. These show the conditions in which general ill health, depression and psychosis should be seen.

ADMISSIONS

Historically, both in Ireland and abroad, Irish rates of schizophrenic admissions to hospitals have been seen as the highest in the world (Cox 1986, Walsh & Walsh 1970). One intriguing statistic was that Irish-born people living in south east England experienced 2.4 times the expected number of admissions for schizophrenia for both sexes. In the Irish Republic, hospital rates were seen as higher still and similarly in Northern Ireland, but markedly less so for Protestants than for Catholics.

The problem breaks down into two related questions: first is the question of madness among Irish immigrants (in this instance, immigrants to England); second is the question of the higher rates among the Irish anywhere and why this is so.

Cochrane & Bal (1987) set out the issues succinctly. They looked at all admissions to hospitals in England in 1981 and found that:

1. the rate of first admission for all diagnoses was more than twice as high for Irish than for English born. For admissions for all diagnoses, rates for the Irish were also much higher than for the English
2. the Irish born of both sexes have very high absolute rates of admission for schizophrenia than the English-born community.

In respect of Irish immigrants, Cochrane & Bal (1987) go on to say that the high schizophrenia rates might be an artefact brought about by demographic differences between the Irish and English and where the link to incidences of schizophrenia is coincidental. They calculated rates for first admissions (of immigrants) and for all admissions and related these to country of birth, diagnosis, age, sex, marital status and whether a first or re-admission. What they discovered was that age was the most significant variable, unsurprisingly since the link between age and schizophrenia is remarkably constant. Schizophrenia tends to occur from late adolescence to early manhood in males, with a slightly higher rate of incidence for females in early middle age. Now, if the age bands of Irish immigrants arriving in England were concentrated in these groups this might account for the higher incidences among them. And this was found to be the case for whereas only 26% of English-born males (in the study) were in the high-risk band (25–44 years), 37% of the Irish born were in this group. For women, whereas 27% of English women were in this group, the figure for Irish women was 52%. The study indicates a need to standardise ages when making comparisons between samples. It was neglect of this variable that had resulted in the earlier skewed conclusions.

However, when direct comparisons are made between Ireland and England, the rates for native Irish are higher than for Irish immigrants; it seems reasonable to conclude, therefore, that the higher rates observed for Irish immigrants are partly accounted for by a high prevalence in Irish people generally. Historically, this has been the sticking point; one could try and account for the increased rates for immigrants in terms of their poor social and economic circumstances were it not for the increased rates in Ireland also.

We need to ask, therefore, why the Irish, wherever they are, exhibit higher rates of schizophrenia. Both for the Republic and Northern Ireland, rates of hospital admissions have been highest in the rural west and declining as one approaches the major towns of the north east such as Dublin and Belfast. The frequency of the illness – sometimes almost double what would be expected normally – suggests, perhaps scarily, a genetic disposition, a belief that gains plausibility as evidence for the biological basis of mental illness gains weight. Against this view is ranked an army of protagonists who insist that social/environmental factors are the fundamental determinant of mental disorder. But whatever the strength of either position – or a mixture of the two – what remains unchallenged is the higher than expected incidence of schizophrenia in rural Ireland.

NEW GROUND

In 1987 and 1990, however, Ni Nuallain et al produced 'breaking new ground' reports which showed incidences to be no higher in Ireland than anywhere else. However, these studies need careful evaluation. The 1990 paper, for example, describes how a Three Counties Case Register had been set up in 1973 (the rationale for this can be found in O'Hare & Walsh (1987)). This register was designed to capture anyone making contact with psychiatric services within this three-county catchment area. Here, Ni Nuallain et al appear to equate 'hospital first admissions' with community prevalence and it is this reliance on hospital admissions to determine prevalence which is risky. The problem is that the Ni Nuallain et al (1987, 1990) studies assume that hardly any schizophrenia lies outside that which is picked up by services. They acknowledge, for instance (1990, p. 138):

> *"We have been unable to take account of people in the community who are not now symptomatic but are known to have been previously ill and who therefore would have qualified for the lifetime prevalence count."*

In addition, underlying these studies lay assumptions that the case register approach recorded no false negatives, i.e. that there were no schizophrenics diagnosed as something else whereas there may well have been.

Conducting research in the same catchment area as Ni Nuallain et al (1990), Torrey et al (1984) noted two consistent findings both for their own and for most other Irish studies. One was that whatever the facts about prevalence rates, poverty was a constant feature in all of those studies. Second was the consistent observation that high incidences occurred within geographical pockets and were not uniform; for instance, Torrey et al (1984) noted that the prevalence rate for one area of County Roscommon was twice the rate found by case register for Ireland as a whole. Both of these indices – poverty and pocket prevalence – impressionistically support Scheper-Hughes' (1979) influential qualitative study (see Ch. 10).

Crucially, the Ni Nuallain et al (1987, 1990) studies also showed that prevalence rates depended upon the diagnostic criteria of schizophrenia employed. Variation in criteria is also evidenced in Torrey's (1987) paper where the enhanced prevalence rates in western Ireland comprised 21 people with DSM-III schizophrenia but also 11 with schizoaffective disorders and four with atypical psychosis. Schizophrenia is not considered by many – not even by conventional psychiatrists – to be a unitary or tight-fit diagnostic construct and Bentall (2004) has shown how the DSM-IV – the standard manual of psychiatric diagnoses – describes schizophrenia in such broad terms as to include practically any odd or unusual behaviour: for example, for those who do not fit its schizophrenia label it has a substitute, 'psychotic disorder not otherwise specified'(!).

Whether or not the Ni Nuallain et al (1987, 1990) findings are sufficient to overturn beliefs about rates of madness that have lasted 200 years is debatable. However, Kendler et al (1993) confirm their conclusions and Ni Nuallain is now the baseline against which all future research should attend.

In the meantime, the question of illnesses unaccounted for by admission rates requires further work. For example, 'the long childhood' of Irish males – those who remain unmarried as they work their parents' farms into middle age – might have afforded 'protection' against diagnoses since such 'children' were generally passive and unlikely to bring attention to themselves. In addition, the reported higher rates among the Irish outside of Ireland also need to be balanced against the newer findings of low prevalence within Ireland. In particular, Cochrane & Bal's (1987) findings in respect of the demography of age are a starting point here. An important factor in this will be the kinds of research that are deployed; probably those that will carry most force and lead to the overthrow of myths and suppositions will be of a statistical demographic nature.

References

Amis K 1991 Memoirs. Penguin, Harmondsworth

Balarajan R, Yuen P 1986 British smoking and drinking habits: variations by country of birth. Community Medicine 8(3):237–239

Bentall R P 2004 Madness explained: psychosis and human nature. Penguin, London

Bolger D 2005 An Irishman's diary. The Irish Times, November 24th

Butler R 1994 Forgotten figures: mental health and the Irish in Britain. Openmind 70:16–17

Cochrane R, Bal S 1987 Migration and schizophrenia: an examination of five hypotheses. Social Psychiatry 22:181–191

Commission for Racial Equality 1997 Irish in Britain. Commission for Racial Equality, London

Cowley J J, Simmons S 1992 Mental health, race and ethnicity: a retrospective study of the care of ethnic minorities and whites in a psychiatric unit. Journal of Advanced Nursing 17:1078–1087

Cox J 1986 Transcultural psychiatry. Croom Helm, London

Davey Smith G 1997 Notes accompanying Nazroo J W 1997 The health of Britain's ethnic minorities. Policy Studies Institute, London

Department of Health 1993a The health of the nation: accidents. HMSO, London

Department of Health 1993b The health of the nation: ethnicity and health: A guide for the NHS. HMSO, London

Department of Health 1996 Patient's charter. HMSO, London

Department of Health 1998 Working together. HMSO, London

Doolin N 1994 The luck of the Irish? Nursing Standard 8(46):40–41

Dunne C 2003 An unconsidered people. New Island Books, Dublin

Fanon F 1986 Black skin, white mask. Pluto, London

Fernando S 1991 Mental health, race and culture. Macmillan, Basingstoke

Finnane M 1996 Law and the social uses of the asylum in nineteenth-century Ireland. In: Tomlinson D, Carrier J (eds) Asylum in the community. Routledge, London, pp. 91–110

Gerrish K, Husband C, Mackenzie J 1996 Nursing for a multi-ethnic society. Open University Press, Buckingham

Greenslade L 1992 White skin, white masks: mental illness and the Irish in Britain. In: O'Sullivan P (ed.) The Irish world wide: history, heritage, identity. Vol. 2. Leicester University Press, London, pp. 201–225

Kelleher D, Hillier S 1996 The health of the Irish in England. In: Kelleher D, Hillier S (eds) Researching cultural differences in health. Routledge, London, pp. 103–123

Kendler K S, McGuire M, Gruenberg A et al 1993 The Roscommon family study I: methods, diagnosis of probands, and risk of schizophrenia in relatives. Archives of General Psychiatry 50(7):527–540

Lee B, Syed Q, Bellis M 1998 Improving the health of black and ethnic minority communities: a north west of England perspective. The University of Liverpool, Liverpool

Littlewood R, Lipsedge M 1982 Aliens and alienists: ethnic minorities and psychiatry. Unwin Hyman, London

Mac an Ghaill M 2000 The Irish in Britain: the invisibility of ethnicity and anti-Irish racism. Journal of Ethnic and Migration Studies 26(1):137–147

MacGiollabhDin P 1995 The Irish in Britain and the psychiatric system. Asylum 9(6):21–23

Marmot M, Adelstein A, Bulusu L 1984 Immigrant mortality in England and Wales 1970–1978: studies in medical and population subjects. HMSO, London

Murphy K, Macleod Clark J 1993 Nurses' experiences of caring for ethnic-minority clients. Journal of Advanced Nursing 18:442–450

Nazroo J Y 1997 The health of Britain's ethnic minorities. Policy Studies Institute, London

NHS Executive 1999 Patient and public involvement in the new NHS. NHS Executive, London

Ni Nuallain M, O'Hare A, Walsh D 1987 Incidence of schizophrenia in Ireland. Psychological Medicine 17:943–948

Ni Nuallain M, O'Hare A, Walsh D 1990 The prevalence of schizophrenia in three counties in Ireland. Acta Psychiatrica Scandinavica 82:136–140

Nursing Times 2000 Call for chief nurse for ethnic minorities. Nursing Times 96(16):4

Office of Population Censuses and Surveys 1991 Census general report. HMSO, London

O'Hare A, Walsh D 1987 The three county and St. Loman's psychiatric case registers 1974 and 1982. Medico-Social Research Board, Dublin

Owen D 1995 University of Warwick Centre for Research in Ethnic Relations/National Ethnic Minority Data Archive 1991 Irish Born People in Great Britain. Census Statistical Paper 9

Policy Studies Institute 1997 Notes accompanying Nazroo J W 1997 The health of Britain's ethnic minorities. Policy Studies Institute, London

Sashidharan S P, Commander M J 1998 Mental health. In: Rawaf S, Bahl V (eds) Assessing health needs of people from minority ethnic groups. Royal College of Physicians and Faculty of Public Health Medicine, London, pp. 282–290

Scheper-Hughes N 1979 Saints, scholars and schizophrenics. University of California Press, London

Tilki M 1998 The health of the Irish in Britain. In: Papadopoulos I, Tilki M, Taylor G (eds) Transcultural care: a guide for health care professionals. Quay Books, Salisbury, pp. 125–151

Torrey E F 1987 Prevalence studies in schizophrenia. British Journal of Psychiatry 150:598–608

Torrey E F, McGuire M, O'Hare A, Walsh D, Spellman M P 1984 Endemic psychosis in western Ireland. American Journal of Psychiatry 141:966–970

Walsh D, Walsh B 1970 Mental illness in the Republic of Ireland – first admissions. Journal of the Irish Medical Association 63:365–370

12 So you think you're funny?

Many a true word is spoken in jest

(Chaucer 1390)

According to Plato, Hobbes, Descartes, Schopenhauer and Freud, jokes are a serious business. This chapter is about the role they play in the perception of Irish people, including Irish immigrants to Britain. I will explore antecedents to the Irish joke critically aligning these with Franz Fanon's concept of dispossession, immigration and self-disgust. The various effects of jokes, for example that the ethnic joke is banal and inoffensive, holds little water with me. In my view, jokes are mechanisms of censure and I cite their ubiquity in culturally dominant contexts as evidence for this.

Adopting facile ideas about other people's cultures is problematic. There is a well-established tradition of writers acquiring a modest acquaintance with Ireland as a prelude to making quite magisterial pronouncements and assessments about it. Herr (1995, p. 276) notes that most outside commentators, at some point, begin postulating traits as a prelude to defining the 'Irish mind' or 'Celtic consciousness'. Perceptions of a carefree, jovial people can turn to notions of Celtic whimsicality – a sort of 'Finian's Rainbow' replete with song, dance and 'the blarney', conceptions of a people detached from secular thought. This dreaminess, in turn, links into a fatal divisiveness, psychological oscillations induced by rapacious religion, rural isolation and converting to 'dispersion and disconnection', not just intellectually but emotionally as well. Hence, the capacity of the Irish joke to narrow the image of Irishness as inferior, as second rate, its ability to framework its target as figures of fun and ridicule. The process is not new:

> *"Most middle and upper-class Victorians preferred to see Paddy as a bundle of Celtic contradictions: a creature both happy and melancholy, drunk on whiskey and drunk on dreams, violent and gentle, lazy and capable of working like a black, ignorant and cunning."*

(Curtis 1971, pp. 94–95)

Accompanying this (supposed) predilection for custom and reverential religion is a strong 'sense of place' (but not identity) and a 'funerary' attitude born of fatalistic obsessions with ill health.

SUPPOSITIONS

Making sense of these suppositions is difficult, hence the slide into simplistic, causal connections between culture and behaviour. However, something considered only rarely within Irish contexts is the conquest of one culture by a dominant other by means of cultural imperialism. Foucault's (1971) concept of discourse, be it about sexuality, madness or culture, determines how things are meaningfully discussed. Drawing from Foucault, Edward Said's *Orientalism* (1978) shows how 19th-century western scholarship came to define the Middle East as 'Other': that is, a supposedly disinterested scholarship rendered another culture inferior by showing that culture as not possessing western sensibilities. It's not that this scholarship establishes 'the truth' of the inferiority of the 'Other' as much as it asserts *itself* to be true; there is only imperial truth and, in an Irish context, primitiveness and rebellion become mirror images to a superior English civilisation.

The plethora of anthropological studies in Ireland during the mid 20th century constituted a discourse about Irish people as defective, which defectiveness flowed from intellectual inferiority. Constructing 'otherness' is not, therefore, a one-off event but a sustained accumulation of positioned truths about the target group. In this instance, inferiority is encapsulated within jokes but takes its strength from derogatory discourses that are much older.

CONSEQUENCES

In respect of the complexity of the jokes' origins, it may help to look at the ideas of Franz Fanon (1986) – a black Algerian psychiatrist – which lend themselves to the analysis of oppressed cultures, especially the manner by which oppression affects mental health. In an Irish context, Greenslade's (1992) reading of Fanon is that, by whatever means colonised peoples cope with inferiority, it becomes particularly difficult for them to do so as immigrants in the country of their perceived oppressors. Although Fanon judges the western/capitalist oppression as having evolved from black Atlantic slavery, his descriptions of immigrant worthlessness apply generally. And, as we shall see, degrading the Irish to a subhuman plateau became a prerequisite by which their 'sufferings' (famine, poverty, death of the language) were belittled and made fun of. Immigrant status confirms worthlessness, provoking the timidity that loss of identity brings. It is at least plausible, given Fanon's 'conditions', that worthlessness may proceed to depression. Equally, if the basis of psychosis is fragmentation, then the Irish immigrant (to Britain) is vulnerable: not wishing to become British, but ashamed of going home, he/she holds to the uncertain hope of going back anyway. This is easily forgotten – that most migrants of whatever origin have little intention of remaining:

> *"Most of the pre-1962 migrants were single men, who usually came with only a short stay in mind: a working trip to Britain becoming an established rite of passage for young men in the Commonwealth, a duty they owed to their families and villages."*

(Winder 2004, pp. 285–286)

Certainly, duty to family and village will ring bells for Irish migrants as well as the money orders posted home, perhaps the unifying factor of immigrants to Britain all told. Also, we are discussing here the Irish poor (of the period) and not:

> *"The successful Irish, the witty Irish, the ambitious Irish, the entrepreneurial Irish, the thrifty Irish do not count, truly as Irish."*

(Winder 2004, p. 163)

Ignoring this can lead one to view all emigration as nasty, degrading and fatal. While true for many, not all carried baggage of poverty, degradation and depression. Nevertheless, significant numbers of immigrant Irish to Britain would soon exhibit high levels of physical and psychological distress (Cochrane & Bal 1987, Finnane 1996) which, till recently, remained hidden. There are various reasons for this. Many Irish are reluctant to see themselves as an 'ethnic minority'; are they not, after all, inheritors of proud Celtic traditions, the progeny of 'the land of saints and scholars'? Consciously dispossessed of this, some may seek to identify with the dominant group and thus avoid exposure as needy and/or demanding, which might draw even more prejudice. It is the configuration of this prejudice as jocularity which concerns us: we must unearth its hidden designs. You could, alternatively, hold that jokes are unimportant, a bit of a laugh, really. Their roots are as follows.

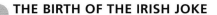

THE BIRTH OF THE IRISH JOKE

In the 12th century, Gerald of Wales (1894, pp. 125–126), comparing the Irish to the Normans, opined that the former live like beasts, a filthy people, wallowing in vice, incestuous, barely human:

> *"This people, then, is truly barbarous … as they inhabit a country so remote … forming as it were another world and are thus secluded from civilized nations, they learn nothing, and practise nothing but the barbarism in which they are born and breed and which sticks to them like a second nature."*

Having slaughtered everyone in the town of Drogheda, God's own ambassador, Oliver Cromwell, wrote:

> *"It hath pleased God to bless our endeavours in Drogheda … the enemy were about 3000 strong in the town … I do not think 30 escaped with their lives. Those that did are in safe custody for the Barbados. I wish that all honest hearts may give the glory of this to God alone, to whom indeed the praise of this mercy [my emphasis] belongs."*

(Downing 1980, p. 13)

Many English writers (for example, Coleridge, 1722–1834, and Spenser, 1552–1599) visualise English civilisation based on laws, versus Irish barbarism based on local kinship, loyalty and sentiment (Deane 1983). To the English, the Irish mind is resolutely criminal with remarkable disrespect for English laws and so for 'the Law' as such. The stereotypes – quaint Paddy or the simian terrorist – arise quite naturally from 19th-century beliefs that criminal types are always identifiable to decent citizens.

In 1836, Prime Minister Disraeli summarised this state of affairs:

> *"The Irish hate our order, our civilisation, our enterprising industry, our pure religion. This wild, reckless, indolent, uncertain and superstitious race have no sympathy with the English character. Their ideal of human felicity is an alternation of clannish broils and coarse idolatry. Their history describes an unbroken circle of bigotry and blood."*

(Kearney 1985, p. 7)

Thus, the Victorian image of the Irish was of a people barely transformed from ape status. The cartoonist Tenniel (of *Alice in Wonderland* fame) forged this imagery in *Punch* magazine where it played a significant role in the emergent concept of 'bogtrotter' or 'thick paddy'. The importance of the animal imagery was that it was seen to underpin resistance to British rule and, indeed, visualising 'the paddy' as part ape, part idiot was consistently paired in cartoons with Fenianism and rebellion. Without doubt, the advent of Darwinism bolstered such thinking. For:

"What was relatively new about the simian image of Paddy was not the sense conveyed thereby of Celtic inferiority and Anglo-Saxon superiority, but rather the scientific impulse behind that image."

(Curtis 1971, p. 99)

It was during this period (about the 1860s), when knowledge of the great apes was disseminating in journals, magazines and newspapers, that the simianisation process proceeded apace. By 1860, Charles Kingsley was calling the Irish 'white chimpanzees' (Kearney 1985, p. 7). Mused Kingsley: 'One would not feel disgust quite so much if they were black: but that they are white-skinned is especially repugnant since it makes them look like us'. Together with Elizabeth Gaskell, Thomas Carlyle preached the idea of a less evolutionary developed race. And it is this defamation of Paddy as stupid which primes the Irish joke. Quintessentially denoting its target as intellectually witless, the joke becomes an imperial tool whereby the teller (and his audience) acquire superiority relative to the joke's subject. This 'Nigrescence' of the Irish was to set them apart from the British 'race'. In addition to stressing biological differences, Childs & Williams (1997) note also that characteristics of nationalism, language (including accent) and religion were also important reasons for disapproval.

THE ELITE

One's audience, its size and composition, matters. The ape cartoons in *Punch* magazine were directed at those who could also read; in contemporary Britain, audiences are limitless and sensibilities more sensitive. The prime-time television audience requires a menu that will not tax its moral sensibilities: political correctness rules. This means reducing levels of crudity (in the case of Bernard Manning, the crudity levels staying high means exclusion from telly land). Actually, verbal humour increases during periods of liberality. As Freud noted, 'Brutal hostility, forbidden by law, is replaced by verbal invective'. Further, the spectacle of ethnic groups laughing at themselves is taken as evidence of the inoffensiveness of jokes.

Since everyone is involved in the joke so must it possess equivalent cultural/political status. Now and then, this 'equivalence' is accentuated when the jokester relegates the dominant group to a subservient role. Bernard Manning, for instance, tells a 'joke' where a 'true' Englishman stands in pouring rain waiting for a bus to take him to the dole queue while a jovial Asian shopkeeper airily waves at him from the upstairs window of his money-making shop. Manning's joke is an exemplar of what Douglas (1975, p. 102) calls the joke as 'an anti-rite' where celebrating dominant values can be just as well achieved while seeming not to be.

SUPERIORITY THEORIES OF THE JOKE

Superiority theories – closely associated with Hobbes (1840) – suggest that we laugh at the pratfalls of others because this enhances our position over them. Freud (1960), alternatively, provides a ropes and pulleys explanation whereby repressed emotions are released via laughter, thus ensuring a saving on psychic energy. If we put Hobbes and Freud together (following Arthur Koestler, 1964) this produces an incongruity theory where the simultaneous perception of a single item within two cognitive frameworks gives rise to the joke. In plain English, both the reduction in tension and the sense of superiority incorporate the contradiction that gives rise to the joke. We laugh not so much at misfortune as at capriciousness; laughter lessens apprehension that similar calamities will happen to us.

Freud also discusses the purposes of jokes (1960, p. 97):

> *"It is either a hostile joke serving the purposes of aggressiveness, satire or defence or an obscene joke serving the purpose of exposure."*

What Freudian theory doesn't explain is why racial minorities sometimes share the joke. Wilson (1979, pp. 218–225) summarises studies which show how ethnic groups accept the stereotyped imagery ascribed to them through jokes. He also notes that the Irish not only tell jokes about themselves but are better at it than most! For Oring (1992), this 'sharing of the joke' contains elements of masochism although a 'psychology of inferiority' seems a preferable concept given that the overriding characteristic is unworthiness. Masochism implies enjoyment (of sorts) whereas sharing jokes can service several needs. Whereas self-laughter anticipates and deflects derision it also imposes a sense of one's self as 'other'. This self-laughter, issuing from psychological uncertainty, is exacerbated by cultural dislocation which stems from emigration. Although such dislocation may provide space for creativity – Edna O'Brien (1963) in England, for instance, or Frank McCourt (1997) in America – its downside is a descent into self-caricature or even madness. However, even here, people deal with caricature in subtle and creatively defensive ways. For instance, Wilson (1979) thinks that individuals may genuinely share the stereotypical put-downs of their group but exempt themselves by criticising those within the group who appear to give the group a bad name. This phenomenon is well established among ethnic groups and is sometimes identified as self hatred:

> *"Beginning with ... Mead's idea of the 'looking glass self' social psychology has assumed that one's self image derives from ... how one is viewed by others. When these views are negative people may internalize them resulting in ... self hatred. This theory was first applied to the experience of Jews but was also soon applied to the experience of African-Americans by ... Franz Fanon ... and others."*

(Steele 1999, p. 44)

The concept may now be extended to divergent subgroups within the Irish population overall, resulting in tensions in terms of how one's group is judged from without.

DIFFERENT STROKES

In the case of the Irish, the superiority jokes of the host (British) group include an element of fear (and loathing). Transforming this loathing to jokes rationalises a crisis between the Irish and 'the British' that few English people comprehend. The Irish joke sustains perplexity at an Irish refusal to assimilate a British worldview. However, prejudice, even when emotionally violent, can entail considerable differences in beliefs about how things are constituted. Thus are the Irish conceptualised as good at colourful stories (the gift of the gab), puckish but morose, a myth-prone race, full of dance (Mary Hickman (1989) observes that the success of *Riverdance* was partly predicated on the surprise effect of its technical virtuosity), charm and chicanery (the blarney) but not given to methodical discourse, not renowned for mathematics, science or philosophy. Historically, these ideas carry such weight that they have the feel of truth about them and, even now, can be difficult to refute if one's starting point is a sense of inferiority. Taking a different tack, Davies (1982) says that emigration invokes anxiety and uncertainty because of having to engage with a new rationality and bureaucracy.

Failure to keep abreast must mean that you lack cleverness and the jokes become a result of this but, as well, a means by which the indigenous population structures and makes sense of this.

ABUSED WORDS

Currently, the three most abused words in the English language are 'just', 'only' and 'some'. 'But Dad, it's just two pounds' comes to mind. More seriously might be: 'What do you mean, you're offended? I was only joking'. Or: 'Honestly, you people just can't take a joke'. Best of all: 'Some of my best friends are Irish' (substitute black, Jewish, Pakistani as required). Well ... it isn't just a joke, it's never just a joke; it's deadly serious and it takes joke form because ape similes would be unacceptable. Not to worry: Irish jokes achieve the same ends as ape similes, only smugly and in relative safety. Jokes, therefore, are always strategic and inherently territorial. Jokes act to gather information in the form of responses (eliciting agreement via laughter, for instance) and can be disowned where they fail to do this. For Goffman (1967), jokes establish boundaries by enabling dominant groups to carve out their turf.

Some argue that jokes are benign. When Travis (1994) interviewed well-known Irish people, for example psychiatrist Anthony Clare, the latter expounded: 'Humour is one of the least damaging ways of expressing aggression. Yes, jokes about the Irish stray away from humour and become something else. But so do Jewish jokes and other jokes ...'. Said Edna O'Brien (1963): 'I'm all for jokes – Oh, let's have jokes. I don't care if they're Irish jokes, Jewish jokes or Siberian jokes. I follow Dr. Johnson's saying: "A man's intelligence can be judged by the frequency of his mirth," wasn't it? I think that sums it up.'

However, whatever predicates are ascribed to jokes, Smith (1996) states: 'We must recognise a difference of interests and see that some parties to the laughter (e.g. the objects of contempt or derision) may not find the joke funny'. Perhaps had Travis asked ordinary people and not famous ones, he might have elicited different responses. In fact, 70% of Irish people living in Britain regard Irish jokes as offensive and oppressive (Commission for Racial Equality 1997).

NOT INFERIOR PER SE

In his *A History of the Arab Peoples* Albert Hourani (1991, pp. 300–301) says:

> *"Defeat goes deeper into the human soul than victory. To be in someone else's power is a conscious experience which induces doubts about the ordering of the universe, while those who have power can forget it, or can assume that it is part of the natural order of things and invent and adopt ideas which justify their possession of it."*

In an Irish context, jokes are a mechanism of dispossession. Endlessly reviled as comical figures and with vulnerability riding on rootlessness, the stereotype cleverly moves from a visual (simian) to a verbal (jocose) depiction; the latter allows for bits and bobs to be added to the joke in terms of who is listening. 'Present company excluded', for instance, permits a) the telling of the joke, b) an observation of its effects followed by c) a relocation of the joke elsewhere. Freud (1960, p. 103) describes it thus:

> *"By making our enemy small, inferior, despicable or comic, we achieve in a roundabout way the enjoyment of overcoming him. A joke will allow us to exploit something ridiculous in our enemy which we could not, because of obstacles in our way, bring forward openly or consciously."*

The wheel comes full circle with the advent of Irish racism and the re-routing of jokes by the Irish towards others. Lentin (1999) recalls a joke told to a customer by a Dublin barber. An Irishman, a Scotsman and a Cuban are travelling by train. The Cuban smokes only half his cigar and throws the other half out the window. Appalled at this, the other two protest but the Cuban says that there are so many cigars in Cuba this is normal behaviour. You're right says the Scotsman: you know, we have so much whisky in Scotland we drink half and throw the rest down the sink. Indeed, you're right says the Irishman: we have so many Romanians in Ireland, we keep some and throw the rest out of the country. Lentin states that the barber couldn't understand his customer not laughing and she quotes Homi Bhabha (1998, p. xvi) that:

> *"joke-work explores the dream's central mechanisms – condensation, displacement and indirect representation – in the quotidian context of communal utterance, making it possible for us to hear the Unconscious speak in the psychopathology of everyday life."*

Lentin (1999) seeks to extend Bhabha's ideas on Jewish self-critical jokes, arguing that racist jokes are revealing not just about their 'victims' but also about those doing the telling:

"Late 1990s 'jokes' about 'throwing Romanians out' make it possible to hear the unconscious speak in everyday language by echoing earlier days when Irish people were not welcome in … the countries of their diaspora."

As well as projecting anxieties onto minority groups jokes accelerate one-upmanship. Let others carry the ethnic can for a change; its Ireland's turn to name the discourse, to talk the talk.

WHAT JOKES ALSO DO

We may ask: why does racism need jokes? In a way, we have answered this: 'successful' racism requires adulteration if it is to work within politically correct situations. Jokes are 'the velvet glove' of racism, a way of making racism palatable, of rendering it unthreatening. Under the mantle of comedy, racism becomes ubiquitous and ubiquity implies harmlessness. I can hear in my head as I write this: 'Oh come on! It's just a bit of fun. Don't be so pompous. You know your trouble? You can't take a joke'.

CODA: THE RULES OF JOKE TELLING

For those who may wish to try their hand at ethnic jokes, the following rules (after Cohen 2001) may help. In matters of joke telling, however, things are rarely black and white and caution is urged.

1. Remember that jokes work not because they tap into truths about their targets but rather because they vitalise truths about how the target is thought of.
2. You must presume that your audience has knowledge of the target, but possibly of precious little else.
3. Be wary: there is no way of gauging the relative offensiveness of jokes.
4. An essential feature of jokes is that they must carry few instructions on the characteristics of their targets: for a really good effect, you should presume your audience already possesses this.
5. Keep your joke precise: 'brevity is the soul of wit'. Given 3 and 4 above, you can assume that your audience will be capable of supplying background information.
6. If you have the slightest doubt about the moral suitability of your joke, do not tell it.
7. Do not unduly worry about 6 above: such doubts are rare.
8. Always use key words such as Paki, Mick, Wog, Wop and so on: these will show that you are in command of your subject.

9. Make it absolutely clear that some of your best friends are from one of the groups listed in 8 above.

10. Seize upon any physical attribute of your target: this will lend authenticity to any attendant psychological insights you might apply.

References

Bhabha H 1998 Anish Kapoor. The Gallery, London

Childs P, Williams R J P 1997 An introduction to post colonial theory. Prentice Hall, London

Cochrane R, Bal S 1987 Migration and schizophrenia: an examination of five hypotheses. Social Psychiatry 22:181–191

Cohen T 2001 Jokes: philosophical thoughts on joking matters. University of Chicago Press, Chicago

Commission for Racial Equality 1997 Irish in Britain. Commission for Racial Equality, London

Curtis L P 1971 Apes and angels. David and Charles, Newton Abbot

Davies C 1982 Ethnic jokes, moral values and social boundaries. The British Journal of Sociology 33:383–403

Deane S 1983 Civilians and barbarians. A Field Day Pamphlet No. 3. Field Day Theatre Company, Derry

Douglas M 1975 Implicit meanings: essays in anthropology. Routledge, London

Downing T 1980 The troubles. Thames/MacDonald, London

Fanon F 1986 Black skin, white mask. Pluto, London

Finnane M 1996 Law and the social uses of the asylum in nineteenth-century Ireland. In: Tomlinson D, Carrier J (eds) Asylum in the community. Routledge, London, pp. 91–110

Foucault M 1971 Madness and civilization: a history of insanity in an age of reason. Tavistock, London

Freud S 1960 Jokes and their relation to the unconscious. Routledge & Kegan Paul, London

Gerald of Wales 1894 The historical works of Giraldus Cambrensis. George Bell, London

Goffman E 1967 Interaction ritual. Aldine, Chicago

Greenslade L 1992 White skin: white masks: mental illness and the Irish in Britain. In: O'Sullivan P (ed.) The Irish world wide: history, heritage, identity. Vol. 2. Leicester University Press, London, pp. 201–225

Herr C 1995 Critical regionalism and cultural studies: from Ireland to the American midwest. University Press of Florida, Gainesville, Florida

Hickman M 1989 The Irish studies scene in Britain: perceptions and progress. In: Irish dimensions in British education. Report on the Sixth Annual National Conference, February 11th Irish Studies Centre, University of North London.

Hobbes T 1840 Human nature: the English works of Thomas Hobbes. Vol. 4. John Bohn, London

Hourani A 1991 A history of the Arab peoples. Faber & Faber, London

Kearney R 1985 The Irish mind: exploring intellectual traditions. Wolfhound Press, Dublin

Koestler A 1964 The act of creation. Macmillan, London

Lentin R 1999 Introduction: racializing the other: racializing the 'us': emerging Irish identities as processes of racialization. Paper delivered at seminar: 'Emerging Irish Identities' at Trinity College, Dublin, November 27th

McCourt F 1997 Angela's ashes. Flamingo Books, London

O'Brien E 1963 The country girls. Penguin, Harmondsworth

Oring E 1992 Jokes and their relations. The University Press of Kentucky, Lexington

Said E 1978 Orientalism. Penguin, London

Smith G 1996 Laughter, footing and the tolerantial self. In: Paton G E C, Powell C, Wagg S (eds) The social faces of humour: practices and issues. Arena Books, Aldershot, pp. 271–296

Steele C M 1999 Thin ice: stereotype threat and black college students. Atlantic Monthly 284(2):44–47

Travis A 1994 Industrial tribunal rules Irish joke racist. The Guardian, June 8th, p. 1

Wilson C P 1979 Jokes: form, content, use and function. Academic Press, London

Winder R 2004 Bloody foreigners: the story of immigration to Britain. Little, Brown, London

Education, education, education

13

A wholly different activity

Experience, the best of teachers

(Weems 1928)

It is regrettable that on the single occasion when a mental health nursing syllabus gave credence to social and psychological concepts of mental disturbance, as well as responses to it, its implementation lasted all of five years. In 1982, the English National Board for Nursing, Midwifery and Health Visiting (ENB) set out a radical prospectus (ENB 1982) whose realisation resulted in courses which, while not eschewing medical concepts of diagnosis and treatment, nevertheless complemented these with material from social, psychological, spiritual and political sources. It says something about the commitment of those whose brainchild the 1982 syllabus was that it quickly perished with the onset of Project 2000 courses in the early 1990s (Le Var 1997a, 1997b). One might have imagined that this syllabus and the many curricula it inspired would have formed a bulwark against external encroachment on psychiatric education and practice. But this was not to be. So how did such an educational coup occur so quickly and effectively? How could the ENB so rapidly accede to an educational hybrid like Project 2000 which, through its 'Common Foundation Programme' (CFP), dispossessed psychiatric nurses of their best chance of building intellectual currency about the philosophy and practice of their care? We will leave to the social historians the task of fully working out why psychiatric nurses lacked the wherewithal to resist the educational blandishments of *Le Projet*; how, despite their reputation as articulate, even voluble, people, they were unable to argue the need for autonomy, self-regulation and curricular control. Partly, the reason lay in under-discussed assumptions about nursing as an intellectual pursuit as well as a raft of philosophical declarations about the uniqueness of nursing and the need to spell this out. Such assumptions carry moral as well as educational/political weight and it is the inherent vagueness of such combinations which renders them a moveable target against which to aim.

To assume that psychiatric nurses would have *wanted* to 'opt out' of Project 2000, of course, is perhaps naïve: the fact is they didn't. It's possible that, at the time, they viewed it positively, particularly its promise to deliver educational parity with other professions. As well, vague promises were made about retaining the 'spirit' of the 1982 syllabus. For example, in 1994, a Mental Health Nursing Review (Butterworth 1994) made reference to the content of psychiatric nurse education within a Project 2000 context. Recommendation 7 vaguely asserted that mental health nursing should retain 'its speciality at initial preparation level' (p. 49). Recommendation 31 more specifically stressed that there be a review 'of the time and emphasis given to each of the four branches within the CFP' (p. 52). While some of this has come to fruition, an overall ambivalence and lopsidedness persist within CFP programmes (see Clarke & Flanagan 2003, Ch. 7) which continue to favour the concerns of adult nurses.

DISSIDENTS

I would like to add my name to the dissident practice (Jackson 1999) of seeking a complete withdrawal of psychiatric nursing from Project 2000 courses and a resumption of direct entry to, and control over, an exclusive psychiatric syllabus. That this will occur anyway seems probable: the recent shortening of the CFP from 18 months to 12 is not, I imagine, the last we have heard of shortening. In addition, from May 2000 reforms were implemented which significantly deviated from some of the original provisions of Project 2000. For example, in addition to CFP shortening, students now had to be provided with CFP clinical experiences that matched their chosen specialty. This has resulted in an absurd situation in which psychiatric students continue to receive theoretical input assumed to be universal while acquiring practical experience relevant to their specialty. In effect, the problem of reconciling a curriculum out of kilter with clinical training is solved simply by ignoring it.

To those who advocate resolving these problems from within the Project 2000 construct, my contention is that the issues are so fundamental (and so obtusely misunderstood by non-psychiatric nurses) that only separation will do. Take but one difference: considerable numbers of psychiatric patients do not *want* to be helped and it requires an act of Parliament (an act that, outside psychiatric contexts, seriously violates civil liberties) to enable compulsory treatment to take place. And this is not something that pertains only to those legally detained. It is a commonplace declaration of professional pride that the majority of patients in our treatment centres are voluntary, that they have sought out or at least accepted treatment without coercion. This self-serving claim is widely misleading with little investigation into the social processes by which people are brought into treatment centres: where the documentation states 'voluntary', this is normally taken as read. But as one-time legal advisor to MIND, Larry Gostin (1977), pointed out: who knows what happens in the sitting rooms of psychologically distressed persons late on a Saturday night in terms of *persuading* them to come into care, *persuading* them that the doctors and nurses mean well? It is this frisson of compulsion which qualitatively differentiates psychiatric from adult nursing. But more so, it is the kinds of discussion that such differences require that inclusion in Project 2000 prohibits; indeed, inclusion in this 'reform' swamped the concerns of psychiatric nurses in two ways. In the first instance, the stress on academia pushed curriculumists to invent even more complex programmes of learning, ultimately leading to modularisation where courses are segmented into manageable gobbets each with their own mini assessment and cut-off point. Of course, this piecemeal approach contradicts claims to treat people holistically. On the one hand students are subjected to educational programmes delivered in disjointed parts, but on the other hand the central assertion is about holism. Modularisation in particular disallows *sustained* discussion about the nature of psychiatric nursing: whether, for instance, the shift to community nursing represented merely the relocation of resources or if it foreshadowed changes in attitudes about how mental illness is conceived and treated. Second, while such discussion has persisted – perhaps in angry reaction to the Project 2000 scheme – in general, the medicalisation of psychiatry proceeded apace, even accelerating with the advent of a vibrant bio-technology. When push came to shove, psychiatric nurses – unlike their midwifery colleagues – did not have the wherewithal to articulate a separate identity for themselves. What remained of their identity was dwarfed by the undue emphasis on adult nursing within courses but also within psychiatric nursing itself, divisions concerning humanist versus cognitive-cum-pharmacological approaches. The wider background to this is the intrinsic interest in, and heavy concentration on, education.

EDUCATION, EDUCATION, EDUCATION

It is education, especially curriculum building, rather than possessing a defined knowledge base, that constitutes the hinterland of most nursing lecturers. As a budding lecturer in the 1980s I was disabused of the concept of 'the teacher' as a font of knowledge: rather was the teacher a facilitator, someone who encouraged students to build up knowledge from what they knew already. Today's nursing students come to know quickly the ritual of being 'broken' into subgroups so as to solve this or that problem while the teacher mysteriously departs the classroom only to return later so as to engage them in a 'discourse' on their findings. When they do teach students on the finer points of empirically derived material this is typically stuff borrowed from other disciplines such as anatomy, ethics, psychology or sociology.

Educationalists are 'when', 'where', 'how' and 'how often' people, becoming slightly uncomfortable if asked to address questions of 'what' is to be taught. If, for instance, you were waiting for an educational authority like the Nursing and Midwifery Council (NMC) to inquire about the *content* of nursing courses you would be waiting a long time. It is hardly surprising, therefore, that nursing courses, and no doubt others besides, emphasise process over substance, conceiving curricula as jigsaw puzzles wherein myriad objectives – by whatever contemporary labels these are known – are matched with ordinary human activities – so as to produce mosaics of learning. In fairness, Project 2000 schemes did invoke holism as an underlying philosophy espousing, at the same time, buckets of rhetoric about person-centred care. But, of course, psychiatric nurses had long since absorbed much of this which meant that they had to watch adult nurses boast their uptake of these as though something new. However, psychiatric nurses' uptake of person centredess was not without interprofessional conflict and this can be a sticking point, trying to persuade non-psychiatric nurses of the ideological differences which still befuddle mental health practitioners. For example, one group (Keltner 1996) has sought to re-establish biology, pharmacology, genetics and medical technology as core elements of the mental health nursing syllabus, their concessions to psychology and sociology affirming the efficacy of cognitive behaviour therapy and other measurable interventions. These elements, in turn, are vigorously objected to by those (Barker et al 1998) who wish to affirm the centrality of patients' experiences and building responses to these in keeping with their (the patients') narratives.

It remains to be seen who eventually will 'prevail' or whether, as Steve Tilley (1998) believes, elements from both will be sustained within an overall setting of varieties of clinical practice. Whatever: it is a debate which is at odds with adult nursing whose educational needs are about acquiring the skills to manage the biological/pathological status of their patients. Although some might protest this, few adult nurses would deny that their work is governed by medical prescription; while they may seek to redress patients' general needs, this hardly detracts from the core determinant which is the patients' medical state. It is simply not true – whatever the jargon of holism – that heart disease is about the 'absence of health'; heart disease is not the absence of anything, it is the *presence* of breathlessness, of not being able to walk, of being in pain, of having a wrecked ventricular wall. Whatever the holistic ambitions of some nurses in pursuance of 'health for all', the heart of medicine and nursing is the treatment of diseases and caring for those who have them. Whereas, in psychiatry, debates which seek to define aberrant behaviour as illness (or not illness) are still viable and continue to take up journal space as well as time on the conference circuit (Bentall 2003, Johnstone 2000).

THE NEW HOLISM

Adult nurses may protest the seriousness of their new-found humanism. However, theirs is a 'phoney war', a war which asserts holistic health care but which ignores the reality of having to work in tandem with medics and in settings whose primary concern is physical ailment. Naturally, this is true for nurses working in psychiatric treatment centres as well: they too incline towards considerations of psychiatric *illnesses* and their medical treatment. However, for some of them, plausible dissension from medical constructs persists: either they wish to imbue psychotic illness with philosophical or social significance or they seek to extend psychological 'care' into everyday problems and personal relationships. This 'debate' – wearying to some – nevertheless has a creative tension which prevents the kinds of moribund practice which theoretical disregard brings. Putting matters bluntly, while many psychiatric nurses accept medical jurisdiction, a dissenting minority – an awkward squad – seeks to prevent practice from sliding into the types of institutionalisation which characterises, especially, long-term care and which has long been associated with medical control (Martin 1984). That the kinds of care that psychiatric nurses now want to deliver are still incompatible with the remnants of our hospital system, and especially acute admissions wards, is now well established (Clarke & Flanagan 2003, Norton 2004).

No greater barrier prevents theoretical growth than the belief that what unites the various branches of nursing outweighs their divergent properties. This is certainly true for psychiatric nursing.

Whether, for instance, paediatric nurses would see their role as qualitatively different to that of their adult colleagues is for them to say; accusations to the contrary (Clarke 1999) await contradiction. Psychiatric nurses *are* different; their historical evolution as an occupation is different, the role of gender in that evolution is very different. Historically, men have played a stronger role in psychiatric nursing so that, for instance, trade union influence was comparatively stronger in psychiatric institutions than in other kinds of nursing. Not that this influence necessarily facilitated good care. Close links existed between unions and nurse managers who had themselves 'risen in the ranks' and who were not well disposed to critique professional working practices. The close (almost symbiotic) liaison between unions and managers, particularly within state (forensic) hospitals, bore directly on the care of patients and the resulting orthodoxy that was largely regimentation and control. When change came, its immediate effect was of increased expectation, even euphoria. However, while the Salmon Report (DHSS 1966) provided nurse leadership with clinical components that might have promoted experimentation of ideas and approaches, it was implemented so quickly that the new 'nursing officers' immediately collapsed into a narrow managerialism from which they, and their successors, never recovered.

SOCIETAL REGARD

Trying to work out society's regard towards psychiatric nursing is not easy; both manifest and submerged notions of madness, and the apprehension that accompanies this, confuse the picture mightily. The element of compulsion and how this is managed is certainly one consequence of societal attitudes. Given that compulsion may be legally sanctioned within community practice, now, more than ever, is there needed some space to discuss these issues and initiate workable solutions to them. But it becomes difficult to discuss whether to define psychological distress as illness where the concerns of adult nurses dominate. Of course, adult nurses will insist that their medical 'attachment' is but a small part of their holistic orientation. Even their most sober commentators (Witz 1994), however, suggest the excessiveness of 'enhanced nursing role' claims, commenting that much nursing activity is still predicated on medical decisions. It's true that medical advocates inhabit psychiatric nursing as well and with an enthusiasm for pharmacology in excess of what one might expect from *any* nurse!

We therefore take comfort that psychiatric service users are rarely enamoured of medical approaches or physical treatments (Coleman & Smith 1997) and place their trust in therapeutic approaches which acknowledge their stories and experiences. Of course, those patients satisfied with medical treatments are less likely to say so. Nevertheless, the meanings of mental distress require broader description than that provided by medicine alone: what it means to experience mental illness within social and economic – especially occupational – perspectives is important. Others will see this emphasis on experience as detrimental (McKenzie 2005), preferring to see nurses acquire skills which can be brought to bear on experience, which is to say, they wish to see the nurse as a *therapist* (MacInnes 2001). However (or even if) these matters are resolved, my feeling is that the energy expended on Project 2000, the endless wading through curricular designing, much of it insisting that mental health components achieve 'parity' with parallel adult content, leaves little time to work out differences. Without the disruption of Project 2000, a more vibrant awareness of the need for psychiatric nursing to construct broader spectrums of community involvement across social, economic, ethnic and gender lines might have ensued.

THE FUTURE

In an English context, change will not come at once but, gradually, eventually, it will come. The *Making a Difference* (DoH 1999) reforms swept away some of the worse excesses of conglomerate nurse education although they did not go far enough. Further change will in addition be piecemeal. However, the end result will contradict the error that the one word 'nursing' conquers all. Psychiatric nursing is qualitatively different to its other forms, so much so that even to continue to describe it as nursing seems puzzling. If you were to proffer descriptions of adult nursing, its psychiatric variant and social work to someone ignorant of any of these, it seems difficult to imagine them having trouble separating the first two. However, determining where the latter two begin and end might prove a more difficult proposition. Of course all of this discussion presupposes, somewhat, that adult nursing is capable of defining itself but this too is not so; were it so, then it would do it satisfactorily. The only way open for adult nursing to do this is to concede its close connection with medicine. Adult nurse spokespersons are reluctant to do this because of the possible negative implications for professionalism and equal standing. They have opted conclusively for holism and those features which they believe to be endemic to nursing full stop. But it is this ecumenism, embodied within Project 2000, that makes it difficult for psychiatric nurses to disentangle themselves and go home. That, of course, begs the question of where home is and while ideological rifts continue to identify subgroups as different as chalk and cheese – the differences are not just window dressing or issues of emphasis – it may be difficult to formulate policies and positions acceptable to all. If one examines, for instance, those psychiatric nurses who seek collaborative approaches with psychiatrists and other medicalists this presupposes agreement with medical explanations of mental distress. Contrast this with something like the 'tidal model' (Barker & Buchanan-Barker 2005) and one faces a difference of colossal proportions. One solution would be to concede that nursing is linked to medical practice and that its utter dissimilarity to something like the tidal model means the latter could secede from nursing altogether. That it doesn't do so, or finds it impossible to do so, can only be as a result of a perceived unifying quality of caring, a nursing attribute that is conceptually losing ground by the minute.

References

Barker P, Buchanan-Barker P 2005 The tidal model: a guide for mental health professionals. Brunner-Routledge, Hove

Barker P, Reynolds W, Stevenson C 1998 The human science basis of psychiatric nursing. Perspectives in Psychiatric Care 34:5–14

Bentall R 2003 Madness explained: psychosis and human nature. Penguin, Harmondsworth

Butterworth Report 1994 Working in partnership: a collaborative approach to care. Mental Health Nursing Review Team. HMSO, London

Clarke L 1999 Spare the rod – protect the child. Paediatric Nursing 11(3):6–9

Clarke L, Flanagan T 2003 Institutional breakdown. Academic Publishing Services, Salisbury

Coleman R, Smith M 1997 Working with voices: victim to victor. Handsell Press, Runcorn

Department of Health 1999 Making a difference. HMSO, London

Department of Health and Social Security 1966 Salmon Report. Report of the Committee on Senior Nurse Staffing Structure. HMSO, London

English National Board for Nursing, Midwifery and Health Visiting (ENB) 1982 Mental Health Syllabus. ENB, London

Gostin L 1977 A human condition. MIND, London

Jackson C 1999 Horses for courses. Mental Health and Learning Disabilities Care 2(12):410–411

Johnstone L 2000 Users and abusers of psychiatry, 2nd edn. Brunner-Routledge, Hove

Keltner N 1996 Psychoanatomy of schizophrenia. Perspectives in Psychiatric Care 32:32–35

Le Var R 1997a Project 2000: a new preparation for practice – has policy been realized? Part 1. Nurse Education Today 17(3):171–177

Le Var R 1997b Project 2000: a new preparation for practice – has policy been realized? Part 2. Nurse Education Today 17(4):263–273

MacInnes D 2001 The nurse as therapist and counsellor. In: Forster S (ed.) The role of the mental health nurse. Nelson Thornes, Cheltenham, pp. 64–91

Martin J P 1984 Hospitals in trouble. Blackwell, Oxford

McKenzie R 2005 Am I flogging a dead metaphor? Sloppy scholarship and the implied spider. Journal of Psychiatric and Mental Health Nursing 12:550–555

Norton K 2004 Re-thinking acute psychiatric inpatient care. International Journal of Social Psychiatry 50:274–284

Tilley S 1998 Sustaining varieties of practice. Paper presented at The ENB National Mental Health Conference, Robinson College, Cambridge, June 29th–30th

Witz A 1994 The challenge of nursing. In: Gabe J, Kelleher D, Williams G (eds) Challenging medicine. Routledge, London, pp. 23–43

14

Why is he taking the Mickey?

His had been an intellectual decision founded on his conviction that if a little knowledge was a dangerous thing, a lot was lethal

(Tom Sharpe 1974)

One-time Conservative Party Leader Michael Howard's statement (BBC News 2003) that too many higher education students were doing too many 'Mickey Mouse' courses begs the question of whether he had nurses in mind when he said this. If we imagine that he did, and recognising that nursing is a predominantly female occupation, it may have been more fitting had he pinned his colours on Minnie Mouse and not Mickey. Indeed, isn't this neglect of Minnie yet another example of male ascendancy and female subjugation? Only joking. Yet, the uses to which education are put, the ambitions it serves, can overreach its intrinsic (educational) value. For even if nurse education does not merit university standing, its entry into the college system has enhanced the status of a largely female (and still emergent) profession. Of course, nursing is not unique in this and others – perhaps those whom Mr Howard had in mind – also seek advancement: film studies, media studies, equestrian and tourism studies, all wish to reinvent themselves within the groves of academe.

There used to be but two secular professions that straddled the worlds of academia and practice: medicine and law. My guess is that even these would prefer the practical aspects of the job and not its theory. After all, how much theory is needed to adjudicate the grubby details of acrimonious divorces or administer an injection, the latter a practical skill honed by technique and experience? I injected numerous people with barely a rudimentary grasp of rear-end muscles and sciatic nerves; experience took care of the rest. That said, both legal and medical trainings entail the inculcation of analytical (deductive) reasoning, essential to making diagnoses and a hallmark of professional judgement. While some higher level nursing studies echo this, pre-registration courses do not. But although they lack (and have no need of) the depth of medical training, practical medical skills are still required. It is at this point that students complain that such training is never enough, nor is it compensated for, as they see it, by alternative textbook derivations of psychology and sociology.

THE STUDENTS

For adult nursing students, it is the sociological realm that is the problem. My impression, supported by research (Clarke 1991) as well as discussion with mental health lecturers, is that adult nursing students resent social sciences in their curriculum, craving, instead, 'more A&P' (anatomy and physiology). These resentments suggest that contemporary curricula are out of sync with students' perceptions of their role in the workplace. Few arrive at the nursing institute without preconceptions; many are already socialised into an occupational mindset with which they imbue their student role. No doubt augmented by working in nursing homes or the NHS (via agencies) this mindset determines what they want to learn. When on clinical placements they quickly suss which parts of the curriculum 'fit' and which parts don't. That they become ensnared by the requisites of practice, and to the extent that they do, is problematic. Ensnared may be too easy though: it's possible that they perceive nursing to be part of the real world, a world of common sense and unencumbered by abstract reasoning. Thus the phenomenon of adult students coming to me, tears streaming down cheeks, clutching failed assignments titled: 'Critically Assess the Therapeutic Properties of Transactional Analysis' and exclaiming: 'But I came here to be a nurse!' You cannot but wonder what they have in mind when they say this. Nor is it easy to fathom the putting together of nursing curricula which take little account of how students perceive theory and practice and their beliefs about how these ought to interface. Students face mountains of rhetoric about theory and practice but are advised that whatever the gap between them, it can only narrow through theory taking the lead and not the other way around. One cannot escape the notion that students and the learning process are being used here as 'a means to an end', classroom fodder for an educational elite determined to proselytise 'new nursing' as a means towards establishing equality with more prestigious professions, a determination that would falter were more traditional concepts of nursing allowed their place.

SERIOUS SIDE

It must have occurred to those who 'drove' the 'new nursing' that a reinvigorated profession could not have medicine as its knowledge base since another profession already had it. Yet faced with a changing role, and especially the move into universities, the hunt for a knowledge base that would distinguish nursing from medicine became imperative. In general, combinations of *holism* (whose theoretical foundations Bertrand Russell had shattered in 1946) and *caring* were trotted out as alternatives being shunted into nursing curricula but with little critical attention to their weakness as explanatory instruments of theory or definitions.

If we take caring as a starting point, a more critical approach may help explicate its usefulness but also its weaknesses as a definition. Introducing a concept of caring solved identity problems for nurses and they duly trumpeted it as an ethical and knowledge base for their practice. Caring, however, as Allmark (1995) has shown, is redundant when it fails to state what it is one cares about. Putting this bluntly, I could just as well kill you from a duty to care – not wishing to see you suffer – as intervene to prolong your life; the fact is, I could perform either action from a caring standpoint. You might argue that the Nursing and Midwifery Council's code of conduct's (NMC 2004) stipulation that nurses 'act to identify and minimise the risk to patients and clients' would obviate the need to make ethical decisions at all. However, 'minimising risk' might be conceived of as not allowing someone to suffer unduly; alternatively, for psychiatric nurses, it could mean *taking* risks as an important component of care delivery. In this instance, is allowing greater autonomy to patients a clinical decision or does one owe a duty to the wider public in terms of ensuring its safety? Clinical practice has always distanced itself from the cultures within which it operates, insisting on a scientific objectivity which prohibits interference in socio-political and economic affairs. But this is a smokescreen of sorts: forensic psychiatry, for instance, is intimately involved in judicial detention both passively and positively.

It was the drive for a more prestigious reputation that led to the abandonment of critical reflection, reflection that might have thwarted the contrived schemas of professionalism supported by academia. There cannot, in fact, be an ethics of caring where there is no object to which that caring is directed or applied. One may care passionately for something that is evil as well as good; to that end, critical acuity, over and above a 'caring' impulse, needs to determine what is worth caring about. To assume that nurses – of any stripe – possess 'caringness' either inherently or via its inculcation through 'training' is mistaken especially when history shows that the opposite can be the case. This is not to deny nursing its intrinsic decency or to demonstrate any less a caring disposition than that possessed by others. That said, how wearying must it be for other professionals to listen endlessly to nurses' proprietorial claims on caring. And while holistic thinking has deviated from narrow conceptions of patients' problems towards more comprehensive assessments this does not mitigate its scholastic weakness. This weakness becomes explicit when forced to connect with clinical pragmatism.

And this is where Mr Howard re-enters. The problem is that universities are not places where ideas are reformulated so as to suit clinical need; in the academy, ideas are worked through to their conclusion and for their own sake. Adult nursing needs to show that it does this; medicine and psychology do as does psychiatric nursing when it disputes received ideas about mental illness as it evolves theories of its own. An example of this is the 'tidal model' (Barker & Buchanan-Barker 2005) which divorces psychiatric nursing from positivism towards a position where experiencing illness becomes the determining point of recovery. Adult student nurses, alternatively, seek descriptive curricula, watered down versions of medicine, and they resent being denied them by curriculum developers, academic supervisors and lecturers. This became abundantly clear with Project 2000 which, in its original form, was saturated in holistic and sociologese jargon. It soon became clear that its imposition was unworkable because it was unacceptable to many students. Following several reviews (MacLeod Clark et al 1996, White 1995) its content was gradually brought into line with more realistic ends.

A second dimension to this is that the numbers of adult nursing students must be kept up; recruitment is an issue because general hospitals need nurses. Yet some moral obligation should attend student interviews so as to ensure that only those of appropriate character and ability are selected. Among mental health lecturers, there is concern that the dislike of non-medical subject matter by adult nursing students is compounded by their difficulties in managing conceptual material. In a training context this may be no bad thing and, actually, adult nursing students might better embrace the interpersonal dimensions of their work were it presented to them in more down-to-earth ways, liberating them from the misery of ologies and isms.

SO IS NURSE EDUCATION A MICKEY MOUSE UNDERTAKING?

I wonder what Michael Howard would say? He chose a derisory phrase to make his point and in so doing showed insensitivity towards the broader needs of whomever he had in mind. My guess is that he (and others) probably do see nursing in this way which is that, despite worthy attributes, nursing is misplaced as an academic discipline. That being the case, is this fair comment? At the time when he said it, many thought that it was. For example, sections of the press became convinced that the new 'graduate profession' was a corruption of traditional nursing. Right-wing journalists (Marrin 1999, Murray 1999) insisted that nurses 'get back to the bedside', that matron be brought back, that nurses stop refusing to do the 'basics'. Constant bickering about hospital hygiene ensued whereby other professional groups were curiously exempted, the assumption being that the housework element of hospital life was the prerogative of nurses. These criticisms were unconsciously anti-women, born of dismay that nurses could conceive of their work as not common sense or 'hands on'. If anything symbolised the media's dismay it was their, ultimately successful, campaign to 'bring back matron'. And back she came albeit under different guises which suggested some disquiet about the whole miserable business. There arose some exchanges in the nursing press about the implicit sexism of the title as well as hurried denials by its supporters that it did not herald a 'return to the past'. So-called 'modern matrons' will insist that they be identified as leaders and innovators. Their rediscovery, however, directly stemmed from political demands – I recall Conservative MP Anne Widdecombe being superbly strident – that nurses 'go back to basics'. At best, the co-existence of 'matrons' with 'consultant nurses' (a particular favourite of Tony Blair) suggests ambivalence about what nursing is, what it may become. And now, to add to the cacophony, we are to have 'dignity nurses' (Womack 2006) thrust upon us, nurses whose remit – at sister, matron and chief nurse levels – will be to ensure that the respect and dignity of patients are maintained while the other nurses do what? Still, it's a perception which says that all is not right, that the basic dignities are in some way in neglect.

Some years ago I argued that we should leave aside narrow conceptions of mental illness and its treatment, insisting what much of what was wrong or insufficient about hospital care could be righted by ensuring for patients 'the ordinary decencies of daily life', that there was little need of bloated, self-important nursing models; sufficient unto the day was the common respect and essential politeness that most people expect as a natural right. You do not have to conceptualise dignity: you identify its lack or its absence and respond to that. Nevertheless, there is uncertainty about these things. According to Professor Ian Philp, who wrote the government's report on 'dignity nurses':

"Shouting at patients, failing to ensure that they were properly fed and clothed, or allowing them to soil themselves, would be treated as seriously by health watchdogs as failure to meet waiting-time targets."

(Womack 2006)

It becomes hard to marry up Philp's description with all of the recent trumpeting about the 'new nursing' and its postmodernist underpinnings, and much of the confusion can only stem, in my view, from the basic falsehoods embedded in pre-registration training; the inability of those in positions of influence to take student dissension (and need) seriously. There is a need for psychiatric students to have an exclusive curriculum which provides them with the skills but also the multiple theories which underpin those skills and justify them: a university curriculum which questions, even, the very notion of skills. With the withdrawal of psychiatric education the adult nursing students, by default, will have their own curriculum which can, I think, be fitted around a two-year – non-university – programme which gives them the professional equipment to work competently in medical settings. Of course there also needs to be present awareness of the wider needs of patients, the 'dignity factor' from which much else will flow: rights to information, to choice, to physical and mental comfort, to privacy and so forth.

SUFFICIENT UNTO THE DAY?

Is it right to ask the adult nursing students to withdraw from the universities? Should their training schools be re-aligned with hospital and treatment centres? In my view they should. The fact is, much that concerns adult nurses lies beyond the remit of what universities can do: this is true for others as well. Even the concept of 'university' is now up for grabs since virtually anyone is now eligible to attend. This, of course, is Michael Howard's point and if carried to its conclusion – which presumably it will be when the Tories return to power – should signal the end of 'widening participation' schemes and a redefining of the university in more exclusive terms. Perhaps, though, the horse has bolted and we shall soon be seeing in nursing an 'all-graduate' profession, the endpoint of professional ambition.

FUNDAMENTAL QUESTIONS

Nurse educators need to recognise that an all-graduate profession sits uneasily with the broad base of nurses who see no contradiction, practically or conceptually, in working with and, in medical matters, taking direction from medical colleagues. We have lost the kinds of training that accounted for this relationship and its permutations in treatment settings. The heart of the problem is a fear of 'training' in a culture that places great store by intellect; nursing, becoming infected with the latter, allowed itself to drift from everyday practice. Reconstituting basic training would not mean neglecting analysis or critical thinking but it would relocate these to practical abilities and caring propensities. Others will argue that contemporary nurses must conceptualise about things, must account for their actions by means of rationales and defensible ideas. That, however, requires us to explain how the practically minded have, till now, managed to succeed estimably in practice! Witness, for instance, the anger of one student's mother who wrote how it was:

> *"demoralising [for her daughter] to work alongside those who put no effort in – yet pass assessments/placements."*

(Anonymous 2003, p. 15)

Self-evidently, academic achievement is not a condition of successful practice whatever its advantages may be to advanced practitioners. Yet what constitutes a good practitioner is only answerable within contexts of practice. Further, the problems of pre-registration adult nursing students are not helped by ill-founded beliefs about common elements which conjoin all nursing. In what way exactly are the problems of postsurgical patients the same as those of patients with schizophrenia, some of whom do not *want* treatment? Finally, no shame attaches to being outside the university system. Psychoanalysis has largely operated outside it as indeed has some medical and legal training, not to mention alternative therapies and a host of others. The issue is about suitability in respect of training people to implement the essentials of care and treatment in medical settings. It is about how to construct a balance between the needs of service provision and a curriculum which does this but without foregoing a critical edge altogether.

References

Allmark P 1995 Can there be a science of caring? Journal of Medical Ethics 21(1):19–24

Anonymous 2003 Letters section. Nursing Times 99(15):15

Barker P, Buchanan-Barker P 2005 The tidal model: a guide for mental health professionals. Brunner-Routledge, Hove

BBC News 2003 Howard renews tuition fees attack. Online. Available: http://news.bbc.co.uk/1/hi/uk_politics/3297173.stm

Clarke L 1991 Attitudes and interests of students and applicants from two branches of the British nursing profession. Journal of Advanced Nursing 16:213–223

MacLeod Clark J, Maben J, Jones K 1996 Project 2000: perceptions of the philosophy and practice of nursing. English National Board for Nursing, London

Marrin M 1999 Nurses are the problem. The Sunday Telegraph, January 10th, p. 31

Murray I 1999 Back to the bedpans for student nurses. The Times, January 16th, p. 1

Nursing and Midwifery Council (NMC) 2004 The NMC code of professional conduct: standards for conduct, performance and ethics. NMC, London

Russell B 1946 History of western philosophy. George Allen & Unwin, London

White E 1995 Project 2000: implications for mental health nursing. Mental Health Nursing 15(2):13–15

Womack S 2006 Dignity nurse in every hospital. Daily Telegraph, April 24th. Online. Available: http://www.telegraph.co.uk/news/main.jhtml?xml=/news/2006/04/20/nurse20.xml

15

Putting students (and the subject) first

An ounce of practice is worth a pound of precept

(Old proverb)

In Athens, two thousand years ago, a grotesquely featured teacher – stout, bald, snub-nosed, thick-lipped, protruding eyes – called Socrates wandered the streets perpetually on the lookout for arguments; more often than not he found what he was looking for. Many would rue the day they stopped to discuss the issues of the day with him for he would flummox them with contradictions and put-downs of what, till then, they had believed indubitable. Such teachers especially attract the young, an age group generally unsure of anything but – when appropriately provoked – ripe for debate and intellectual challenge. Sentenced to death by the city authorities (the execution of which sentence becoming the occasion for another Socratic argument!) on charges of refusal to worship the city gods and 'corrupting the young', he was innocent of both charges. That said, a lot depends on how you define corruption and there may well have been a sense in which he was seen as disrupting the body politic insofar as he was leading young men along wayward political paths. As De Burgh (1953) observes, the mystery is why the city politicians waited so long to get him as he had long been a thorn in their side. They trumped up the most plausible charges against him even if, at bottom, his real mistake was to have raised his voice against the political status quo, against them.

THE UNEXAMINED LIFE

Socrates had stated that 'the unexamined life is not worth living' and had set about jolting people out of the complacency of their everyday beliefs. Such challenges to received wisdom or 'common knowledge' are often resisted by the wider population and those who issue them are resented. As a generalisation, and to this day, intellectuals can be viewed with suspicion and especially in some places more than in others. While, for example, France is renowned for its admiration of intellectuals and academics, England, alternatively, is said to be especially suspicious of 'eggheads'. As Jeremy Paxman (1999, p. 188) notes:

> "If you are going to be an intellectual in England, you had better do it discreetly, and certainly not call yourself an intellectual. It does not do to grow passionate about your beliefs or to believe that every problem has a solution. Above all, don't look clever."

Indeed, pushing for alternative solutions to problems – especially where this involves debunking conventional views – can be perceived as fomenting unrest. Greek intellectual life promoted an active interest in one's society and Socrates' 'university' was the marketplace and the everyday concerns of its inhabitants. He really did hold forth in public squares, debating topics in real-life settings and, although he wrote nothing down, Plato's earlier dialogues are said to contain his arguments on a range of issues.

He saw the function of philosophy as a search for truth, unencumbered by considerations of the stability – psychological, social or political – of any individual or group. Teaching and learning were not sedate undertakings; they were not about accommodating received ideas – notoriously, a criticism levelled at nurse education (Robbins Committee 1963) until relatively recently – but instead designed to stimulate alternative answers to questions and problems. As nurses are the new kids on the university block, having entered higher education only 12 or so years ago, it might have been expected that they would experience difficulty acclimatising to less hierarchical, less didactic procedures of knowledge acquisition, that they might have balked at the prospect of managing their own learning. Ironically, however, forces within the universities were already working to compartmentalise knowledge in obedience to externally contrived indices (NMC 2006, QAA 1997) of 'quality' and 'excellence' and nurses have had little problem in living up to this. Specifically, the creation of modularisation led to excesses of curriculum management and control as well as immoderate amounts of time devoted to evaluations of the curricular minutiae of courses. In addition to these new orthodoxies, or, perhaps, as a reflection of them, there took place a massive expansion of higher education with colleges battling to increase their numbers across, especially, vocational and humanities courses. This introduced the phenomenon of huge student numbers moving from classroom to classroom, module to module, assessment to assessment. Add to this a plethora of quasi-government audits such as Nursing and Midwifery Council (NMC 2006) targets and Quality and Assurance Agency (QAA 1997) inspections and the overall effect comes to resemble, weirdly, the worst aspects of the old nurse training schools with their excessive officialdom, regimentation and intolerance towards difference.

A proposed rationale for this is that it heightens educational standards. However, an instrumentalism now exists in education which seeks to link educational processes with tangible economic and politically desired outcomes and one cannot help but surmise that externally imposed objectives support these outcomes. In particular, concern is constantly expressed about the likely benefits of educational change and its consequences for stakeholders, meaning, of course, those paying the bills. For instance, should courses be geared towards satisfying the requirements of health trusts and government departments and, if so, to what extent should independent critical review take a back seat to this? What we have now is an imposition of external controls and validation procedures which have the effect, via endless audits, of stifling learning rather than promoting it. Imposing on the deliverers of nurse education politically driven demands that they satisfy the requirements of quality and assessment exercises can lead to disembodied curricula that miss the real needs of students. Furedi (2004) is especially critical of this audit culture which he sees as data collecting that doesn't just measure, but also radically alters, how educational institutes operate. In terms of nursing, what we are left with are modern-day versions of 'visits by the GNC Inspector' which, in their crude way, cultured the workings of the old nursing schools. Things may appear more sophisticated now but the sense of being on one's guard, of having to perform to criteria that don't *really* represent what goes on, still prevails. What this has given rise to is a constant tinkering with curricula seemingly in the direction of more practical concerns. Indeed, the perception, especially by service delivery managers, that there were growing discrepancies between theory and practice led the NMC to re-focus attention to the tightening up of 'essential skills and competencies' (Nursing Times 2006, pp. 18–19). However, this proceeds so slowly that educationalists – with their curricular fussing and fidgeting – can enjoy the illusion that change comes through them when it mostly comes from service demand.

MODULARISATION

Educational programmes are nowadays packaged as modules – self-contained, self-defined units of study which, combined, are intended to form whole, recognisable, courses of study. Modules do have some advantages: they allow students to 'own' those parts of a course which they have completed, whereas before, students lost what they had done if they opted to leave. Also, modules are transferable: students can carry them forward and restart their courses in another place and at another time. Note, however, the sameness which is implied here: the module is a package which has been hammered out consistent with how it has been hammered out elsewhere. The implication is that knowledge can be broken down into manageable bits designed to 'fit' classroom teaching and this can make the kind of Socratic dialogue – which some would still see as the heart of teaching – fairly redundant. Standardisation of curricula and the nitpicking mechanisms by which they take shape mean that to dissent from the teaching content which they spawn is considered anathema. In addition, teaching styles have become so enslaved to technology that independent thought or intellectual exchange is side-tracked. Having spent years as a teacher, from primary to university levels, Tom Ward (2003, p. 13) returned to full-time education at a 'venerable' British university. To his amazement he found that the drive for quality assurance had led to a travesty of teaching with sessions 'uniformly dull':

> *"What was it that turned my initial enthusiasm into a sense of boredom, frustration and disengagement, surely the three deadly sins of the learning process? It can be summed up in one word: PowerPoint."*

Ward discovered extraordinary dependence on this 'teaching aid' and concluded that it had built up barriers between meaningful engagements of tutors, students and learning. To this can be added an equally heavy dependence on pre-planned teaching based on overhead projections to which the epithet 'death by overhead' is frequently applied by students. It's as if teachers have lost the capacity to trust themselves or their students; it partly smacks of an assumption that questions to which answers cannot readily be found are either not worth the asking or so ill-founded that the Socratic practice of examining questions, and how we come by them, is discarded. We can link diminished concerns about intellect within higher education with the latter's commodification which occurs, principally, through the marketing of modules. This must be properly seen against a background of theoretical shift and, particularly, the emergence of that phenomenon called postmodernism, whose essential thesis is that no one truth prevails. Truth is now defined as discourse, verbal expressions of power acquisition and maintenance.

This differs profoundly from Socratic dialogue where exchanges service the breaking down of proposition and counter-proposition so as to arrive at valid conclusions, whereas postmodernism holds that there are many truths arrived at in different ways and for different reasons. It is a view which has carried significant weight in recent years and many psychiatric nurses now subscribe to it. In general, validating the worth of everyone's view has bred an egalitarianism which extends everywhere but is especially implicated in education. It has spawned the concept of widening the entry gate; the width of that gate is now immeasurable because if what matters, ultimately, is what 'I' say and how 'I' say it then processes of theory and assessment will necessary follow this. Thus have examinations given way to continuous assessment and 'project work'. This is OK, to an extent, but it has been taken too far, its dominant effect being the idea that content should not unduly inhibit *how* students are assessed. Furedi (2004, p. 4) believes that current university managers:

> *"regard the content of culture and ideas with indifference. Their concern is to use culture to achieve an objective that is quite separate from its inner content."*

Thus, for example, do champions of culture link the learning of modern languages with commerce or they prize the acquisition of practical nursing skills at the expense of critical reflection so as to service hospital or other institutional requirements. If knowledge has become an instrument towards other ends, so too have students become a means by which educational institutes achieve those ends and not least by recruiting students in ever-increasing numbers so that educational standards are compromised. With this in mind, Immanuel Kant's dictum to always treat people not as means but as ends is up-ended and the resulting ethical slippage goes unnoticed amid the welter of commercialism and enterprise. And as for 'widening the gap' to more and more students, this only works where culture and learning are made to be what you want them to be. Far from being anti-elitist, promoting policies of social engagement simply puts the cart before the horse: genuine engagement should emerge from below and not coalesce from the promptings of an educational elite. Programmes of inclusion actually bring about sameness and the acquisition of diplomas whose value lies principally in conferring eligibility for entrance to service and recreational industries.

Yet, while misplaced, the desire to 'educate the masses' seems genuine enough and we need to view it against a background of endemic elitism within British education historically as well as the widely held perception of an inadequately educated populace. Indeed, the recent imposition of university tuition fees *doesn't* reflect Furedi's arguments about standardising views or even participation: such fees may work to divert some from entering higher education at all and they certainly don't point to a population having education thrust upon it. However, for those already within the system, there seems little option but to access 'bits' of information more and more tailored to meet the needs of populations and not individuals. The essentials of this are the supplanting of book reading, and the knowledge derived therefore, with material parcelled as 'workbooks' as well as the Internet, in-house computers and other bits of software. It is now possible for a student to traverse an entire degree programme without actually reading a book 'from cover to cover'. No doubt this is conditioned by Internet technology which demands speed of acquisition and response and which is further driven by the economic status of contemporary students who, working to pay bills and survive, are unable to assimilate what hasn't been reconfigured (for them) into more user-friendly chunks.

FREEDOM OF INFORMATION?

In *The Plato Papers* Peter Ackroyd (2000, p. 16) has a fictional, futuristic Plato respond to an inquiry about information in earlier (21st century) times:

> *"You were asking me, were you not, about 'information'? By all accounts it was a very ancient deity. It conferred power on those who worshipped it."*

Here, information is contrasted with knowledge. Whereas information can be acquired from multiple sources, actual knowledge comes through intellectual debate and reflection. Today, we worship information, we have become dedicated trekkers of the information highway. An example of what this can lead to is the students charged with preparing sessions to teach their fellow students. Their first port of call is always the Internet where may be found much that is good but also loads that is rotten. Even if the sources used are reputable, what tends to be produced has a superficial 'holiday rep' quality about it: information retrieved and processed, intellectual spam. How common is it to walk into computer pool rooms peopled by a dozen students with each one locked into their personal terminal – or alter ego – oblivious to others as they blandly siphon off bullets of information. Unsurprisingly perhaps, there occur expressions of dismay whenever this computer-generated information is challenged or contradicted. This drive for sameness operates at different levels and contexts within educational settings. During an 'appraised' teaching session on the topic of developmental psychology a lecturer chose some lines from Philip Larkin's 'This be the Verse' (1974):

> *"They fuck you up, your mum and dad."*
> *"They may not mean to but they do."*

lines which are about the inescapability of ill-judged child rearing. The idea was to provoke discussion before considering more formal texts by Benjamin Spock and Penelope Leach. In the post-session assessment, the lecturer was cautioned that such language was inappropriate in the classroom and should not have been used. It would be comforting to report that the appraiser issuing this caution was 'behind the times', someone, perhaps, who hadn't kept up with current thinking and so on. Quite the opposite in fact. The language, the quirkiness of using such material in a teaching session, rankled someone who was actually a top educationalist. More so had it been misunderstood and such misunderstandings become common where knowledge of subject is replaced by preoccupation with curriculum design and the mad determination to construct bigger and better 'programmes of study'. The point missed is that what matters about such programmes is what goes into them, their content, and how this informs one's thinking about the wider world.

GIVING WHAT IS WANTED

Developing educational courses has become the means by which the needs of internal and external validating agencies may be satisfied: how to make modules more attractive to potential clients; couching things in the language of objectives, outcomes, competencies and, now, proficiencies. In this context, the teacher (previously expert in this or that subject) is transformed to a facilitator and the library is now a 'learning centre'. Teachers now endlessly scheme to find out how better to organise their teaching and ensure its accessible delivery. The current fashion is to put as much information as possible on computer systems which can then be accessed at will. This has its place but it has been overdone. It's not education, education, education so much as curriculum, curriculum, curriculum. Thus the endless educational audits about how something is assessed, in what form and how often. To what extent does it comply with this or that centralised criteria. Curriculum development has become an art form where the issue is never about producing something of interest to be taught (though that will sometimes happen anyway) but more an issue of constructing documents – to be presented to curriculum review bodies – which will satisfy the minutiae of predetermined criteria about what *form* education programmes should take. It's a bit like constructing a Heath Robinson machine: it is extraordinarily intricate and, although improbable, when assembled properly will work with elegance and precision, its function, however, remaining essentially meaningless.

The overall concern is for quality assurance and thus standardisation and while, from a moral standpoint, there is something to be said for egalitarianism it is not conducive to good education above and beyond rote learning. Students need to *feel* that they are valued; they require tutorial support which is intellectually consequential, not on-line support which is impersonal and sometimes downright in error. The then Secretary of State for Education, Charles Clarke (October 2002–December 2004), seemed to outline a technological vision of his own when he railed against non-productive university courses by which he meant courses not allied to business. His view, in a nutshell, was that:

> *"Universities exist to enable the British economy and society to deal with the challenges posed by the increasingly rapid process of global change."*

> (Vasagar & Smithers 2003)

He seemed to imply that aspiration towards knowledge – for its own sake – was wishy-washy and a bit redundant. In nursing, too, we are frequently reminded that some types of research are favoured by government more than others; that inquiries into the nature of what nursing is should take a back seat while nurses equip themselves for 'nurse prescribing' and other medical enterprises. This is not to decry the latter but to point out that discussions of these things ought not to be just the province of journals and conferences. Nurse education, at all levels, needs to free itself from the straitjacket of quality assessments, curriculum equivalence, the technological temptations of PowerPoint and overheads and get back to some of its doubts and uncertainties. Like Socrates, rather than providing answers all the time (or even trying to) we need more room for questioning and exploration. It's not that politics is absent from the curriculum: it is not. It's just that 20 years ago it was there as a word, a starting point. Now it's surrounded by 50 curriculum words which tell it, the teacher and the student what direction to take. Many nursing institutes now employ 'teaching plans', generic templates which prescribe sessions, ensuring that the 'right stuff' is taught and not contaminated by the idiosyncrasies of this or that teacher. And we cannot 'take to the streets' like Socrates; if we did, we would hardly be executed, just taken to a 'place of safety' so as to learn, perhaps, the error of our ways.

References

Ackroyd P 2000 The Plato papers. Vintage, London

De Burgh W G 1953 The legacy of the ancient world. Penguin, London

Furedi F 2004 Where have all the intellectuals gone? Continuum Press, London

Larkin P 1974 High windows. Faber, London

Nursing and Midwifery Council (NMC) 2006 Head Office, London

Nursing Times 2006 Raising the bar. 102(12):18–19

Paxman J 1999 The English: a portrait of a people. Penguin, London

Quality and Assurance Agency (QAA) 1997 QAA, Gloucester

Robbins Committee on Higher Education 1963 Cmnd. 2154. HMSO, London

Vasagar J, Smithers R 2003 Will Charles Clarke have his place in history? The Guardian, May 10th. Online. Available: http://education.Guardian.co.uk/higher/artsandhumanities/story/0,12241,953165,00.html

Ward T 2003 I watched in dumb horror. Guardian Education, May 20th, pp. 12–13

16 Nurses and higher education

You cannot put new wine into old bottles

(Matthew ix, xvii)

In light of the foregoing, the question of whether nurse education should remain within the university system or return to an apprenticeship training becomes apposite. There are several aspects to this. Importantly, what is the role of higher education in respect of practical professions? If nursing is practice based, then should becoming a nurse require university-based programmes or should these be optional? Which is to say, should not pre-registration training be premised on basic nursing requirements, realigned with service provision, and with university education an option for those who want or need it? Further, how does academic education impinge on the professional efficacy of postqualification practice? Also, compared to other occupations and educational developments generally, what would be the repercussions of nurse education re-grading to a training status? What are the implications of political resistance to the 'educating up' of a predominantly female profession.

THE CENTRAL ISSUE

The central issue is whether a university education for nurses is actually appropriate. However, to do justice to this question we need first to examine whether contemporary degrees reflect the standards which pertained when university degrees were a rarer commodity. Traditionally, Britain has tended to restrict the provision of higher education: in the 1860s less than 0.5% of 18 year olds were at college (compared to 2% in Germany). This went up to 4.5% by the 1960s, 15% by the 1970s (including polytechnics) and topping about 30% by the 1990s (Radford 1997). So that, as opposed to the 217 000 in higher education in 1965, by the 1990s it had risen to over 1 700 000, not counting nurses (Walden 1996) and today, as predicted, it stands in excess of 2 000 000 and counting. These figures imply that the meaning of a university career is nowadays different from what it was. No longer is the BA degree the prerogative of limited numbers of largely middle-class adolescents graduating from English literature or philosophy departments. The post-Thatcherite campus is not the rarefied milieu it used to be. For one thing it is more crowded, with its facilities stretched beyond what could have been comprehended even 20 years ago. Universities are under pressure to generate income and this has resulted in the welcome mat being put down for what were once vocational courses and with entrance criteria stretched to breaking point (O'Reilly 1999). Putting the matter crudely, is the transformation of British universities an outcome of 1970s and 1980s consumerist rhetoric, involving diminished standards and less stringent assessments, or does it represent an educational metamorphosis with many more students and subjects now deemed *worthy* of inclusion? This begs the question: 'worthy in whose eyes and for which reasons?'.

There is a snob factor in education whereby some areas of study are seen as more 'academic' than others. There once was an Oxbridge don who used to regularly deride business studies as 'the servile arts', a not uncommon view. However, others see university education as a means of developing critical awareness irrespective of the area of study, that going to college might even entail becoming a 'better' person. In other words, degree-level study is about subjecting what one does to critical analysis; it is about learning to think in a certain way. Such 'analytic' definitions cut across whether this or that subject is a 'proper' object of study. Instead, academia is about coming to terms with a subject, perhaps even with some regard for its occupational or wider social relevance. To that end, many contemporary nurses declare that they no longer work 'in the dark' but, with university-level preparation, are now carrying out their work with greater understanding; in effect, that nursing is no longer merely a practical undertaking but is informed by theoretical and ethical reflection.

One standard text (Tomey & Alligood 2006) describes over 30 different nursing models and theories, all of them worked out fastidiously and at some length. A major objection to which these models give rise is that they are an exercise in self-indulgence; surely any activity that gives rise to an excess of 30 models is perplexed as to what its basic position is. True, related fields such as psychiatry, psychology and sociology can be described from different vantage points but usually stopping at around five or six types and not seriously diverging from basic first principles. Nursing, alternatively, is swimming in models and, while they overlap to an extent, they can differ markedly. Whatever the motivation behind them, it is not unnoticeable that each is aligned with a single progenitor and with some insistence as to its uniqueness in the world. Faced with such a smorgasbord of options what is a nurse to do? It's a virtual beggar's banquet; however, beggars cannot be choosers if what is on offer jars with streetwise claims about what practically works. And this is an important point: that nursing has become too academic, too cut off from its practical concerns, a distance expressed not only by individuals but by government and advisory bodies. For example, the Council of Deans and Heads of UK University Facilities for Nurses (Martin 1999) spoke against separating nursing from higher education and, among other things, they said this:

> *"At least 25% of those recruited to pre-registration courses are from people without GCSEs or A levels, so to argue that people who are not academic are excluded is inaccurate."*

This creates as much confusion as it dispels for if a quarter of recruits are 'not academic' – have no secondary school qualifications – then what are they doing in a university? Exactly what does this imply, if anything, about the changed nature of universities? Coupled with the large increase in numbers mentioned earlier, these factors support the allegation that standards have lowered unless one is willing to make a conceptual leap whereby lowering standards is redefined as broadening the criteria by which we define higher education. This is a difficult circle to square and solutions will follow general political claims about society and people's roles within it. For the past 50 years we have ploughed one egalitarian furrow after another with concepts of meritocracy outpacing elitism and entrenched ownership. However, meritocracy implies difference, both in achievement and reward, and while many might nowadays agree that all should have glittering prizes, at what price when the prizes, in and of themselves, are of little value? When, under the Freedom of Information Act, De Montfort University was forced to release documentation pertaining to examinations and marking, it turned out that they had marked up some pharmacy students' work by as much as 14% in order to turn modular fails into passes. Although internal and external examiners expressed their dismay at what was going on, a spokesperson for the university declared that they continued to have every confidence in the quality and robustness of their courses, staff and students (Baty 2006).

THEORY AND PRACTICE

The Council further stated that nursing has been a part of higher education for 'less than two short years' but that, in keeping with other disciplines like law and medicine, 'it has a long history of criticism about interconnecting practical competence with the critical analysis which must underpin any quality service'. This is disingenuous, though, because theory–practice divides have actually been more conflict ridden in nursing, something patently echoed in many of its debates (Lakeman 1998, McKenzie 2005). In addition, unlike other disciplines, there are some within nursing who question its academic standing as mere posturing (Williamson 1998). While this reflects concern about the nature of what is taught, it also belies the absence of that comfortable self-assurance which other disciplines have about their place in higher education. A pertinent criticism by Menzies-Lyth (1988) is that little suggested that nurses from the 'shop floor' *wanted* Project 2000 even if, according to Le Var (1997a, 1997b), the profession's higher echelons did. These persistent uncertainties underpin such commissions as the Chief Nursing Officer's review (DoH 2006) into mental health nursing and, at a wider level, concerns about standards in education generally (Tomlinson 2002).

WHY NURSES?

It is not unfair to ask whether nurses require a university-level education. But if it's going to be asked of nurses, then there are others of whom it can also be asked. For example, does university education have a role to play in the armed services or the police? The probable answer would be 'yes' but with the proviso of it being an option and geared towards acquiring higher responsibilities. Options, of course, lead to divisions and competitiveness and few professions lack their hierarchies and greasy poles. Some lawyers get to be Rumpole of the Bailey or high court judges; most, however, spend their time conveyancing houses or sorting out messy divorces. Is a degree needed for that? Hardly, for according to my local radio station you can now purchase do-it-yourself packages for divorce, house conveyancing and the making of wills. I am reminded here of Alan Bleasdale's (1982) *Boys from the Black Stuff*, where the main character, Yosser Hughes, desperate for work, greets every working person he meets with the refrain 'Gissa job. I could do that'.

Plainly there are walks of life where degrees are not necessary even if a growing number of occupations are now 'graduate professions'. Clearly also, forms of validation are needed if occupational roles are to be standardised, and it might well appear odd were nurses to opt out of accreditation systems and especially when some other occupations appear even less plausible for inclusion than nursing.

However, matters are made difficult by the tendency of nurses to opt for all-or-nothing solutions to their problems. Hence the push to make nursing an *all*-graduate profession with the concomitant conversion of those whose initial training (state enrolled nurses) had been mainly practical.

There is an overall reluctance to accept a variety of ways by which people might qualify as nurses. Not that multiple or even dual systems would be an easy option. One can imagine the complications arising in a situation where two newly qualified nurses are assessed for a D Grade post. One has qualified via an academic, degree course whereas the other has been prepared at diploma level. All other things being equal, which one is likely to be favoured within a service-driven milieu? The academically prepared newcomer is now entering a profession composed of a system of grades and which takes more account of short-range practice-based achievements than it does of theory-based, long-range courses. Unless these fundamental conflicts in respect of the *lifetime* careers of nurses are resolved, serious contradiction will attend the education of nurses particularly in relation to their practice. In some ways, these contradictions reflect divisions between a university system which has become more meritocratic as against a secondary school system which continues to divide along class, economic and, consequently, aspirational lines. Hence the determination of some parents to bring the two into alignment in respect of their own children and the political fallout which occurs whenever it is suggested that state-funded schools *select* whom they want to teach. This was the breaking point for the climb-down by Prime Minister Blair (Woodcock 2006) on the issue of educational reform: for the socialists in his party, selection was a bridge too far.

One measure of the political and social sensitivity involved here is the way politicians are hounded by a media scrum which, thriving on suspected elitism, pounce each time one of them sends their child to a non-state school. Thus did Dianne Abbott (Rosen 2003) bring the political house down on her head when she sent her son to a fee-paying school having viciously condemned any and every one else who had done the same thing. The education of children is a divisive topic and the division now finds its way into higher education through the newer universities – once called polytechnics – who lead the way in cramming campuses with as many students as they can. These, of course, include nursing students who are now an important source of income. The older universities have, by and large, steered clear of the 'newer subjects' and one wonders why. Is it possible that in the long run a two-tiered system, similar to the United States, will emerge where, in some cases, a university becomes a building with the name 'university' hung over its front door.

DOBSON'S CHOICE

In general terms, the closest that government has come to explicitly addressing these problems was when the then Secretary of State for Health, Frank Dobson (While 1999), expressed scepticism about university status for nurses. To an extent this was slightly unfair since, for instance, at many universities some of the largest cohorts of students are to be found in business studies departments. Now this is interesting because one could equally ask what need of business degrees: surely business is about making profits? Yet one of our most prestigious contemporary degrees is the Master in Business Administration or MBA. Would, therefore, the Secretary of State for Industry feel comfortable asking the business community to give up its 'unnecessary' degrees in favour of a return to assembly line apprenticeships? Indeed, the more you think about it the more unusual Mr Dobson's position seemed. For example, it is now possible to obtain a degree in retail management, in hotel administration and tourism, in fashion and photography and in agriculture. Even among the hallowed denizens of Oxford University, students have for years taken degrees in agriculture and forestry. Does this mean that the successful farmer needs a university education? It is strange that while little or no notice is taken of chiropody or equestrianism as degree-level subjects, Mr Dobson saw fit to question its provision for nurses.

STEREOTYPES

Our stereotypical notions of what constitutes university life are twofold: on the one hand there is the image of layabout students, drinking themselves stupid while soaking up public funds in support of worthless courses. On the other hand lie Cambridge and Oxford: dreaming spires, languid punting down rivers, louche students having one-to-one tutorials with Nobel Prize winners. The latter is a far cry from the concrete campuses of the 1960s which heralded an explosion in educational provision. However, it is the appropriateness of that development overall coupled with the metamorphosis of the polytechnic colleges which need debating; seizing upon one group, nurses, who happen to be struggling towards independence is both opportunistic and limited. The central issue is the extent to which practice-based occupations require the kinds of critical reflection which operate freely within purely academic subjects or whether proportionally more account should be taken of the practical requirements of occupations. According to Mair Fear, a clinical nurse specialist:

"Nurses are now being taught in the academic arena and as a consequence we lost the focus on some of those fundamentals – for example learning what's important for basic hygiene."

(Vere-Jones 2006a, p. 17)

And from Suzi O'Connor, lead mental health nurse, students:

"haven't got the clinical experience they need. I think we have to go back and mix up Project 2000 with the old fashioned training. I think we went too far the other way."

(Vere-Jones 2006b, p.16)

GENDER

As well as the belief that nursing should forego university status is the role that gender plays within that assumption. There is an anti-women element in the manner by which a right-wing press (Johnston 1998, Marrin 1999, Murray 1999, Phillips 1999) moralised (often virulently) that nurses were no longer 'working' and that their entry into higher education was derisory. If nursing was a predominantly male occupation it is unlikely that calls for a return to 'the bedside' – be it a psychological or literal bedside – would have been voiced with such persistence. Nursing has been, especially at the point of delivery, a female preserve and there may be a sense, among its critics, that nurses have 'got above themselves', allowed themselves to drift from traditional beliefs about their 'proper' calling which is nurturing as well as attending to all things practical.

IN THE MEAN TIME

I suspect that the muddled expectations of service managers in respect of newly qualified nurses will continue. Likewise, the issue of what constitutes an appropriate curriculum for university study will continue for some time, although ultimately return to dual or multiple portals of entry seems inevitable. However, the divisions implicit in such developments are the seeds of future internal strife; already we see that more recognition and higher pay are given to 'special nurses'. This begs the question of what is special about them other than that they populate intensive and high-tech *medical* settings? It is an irony that while major changes in nurse education were premised on preparing practitioners for primary health care practice, the Butterworth report (1998) noted that Britain still prepared most of its nurses to work in hospitals in opposition to a string of policy forecasts which pointed towards a health care system with primary care at its base.

At the same time, can any economy sustain the kinds of salaries which, historically, have been associated with the classic professional groups if there is added to the fold a more densely populated profession like nursing? Is an all-graduate nursing profession, in this financial sense, possible? If not, then this factor alone will ultimately decide many of these questions, for example the selection of limited numbers who will do the 'nurse' prescribing and perform other specialisms, bear the title 'consultant nurse' and so on. In the meantime, the broad mass of nurses must ponder the moral rightness of their claim to professional status against the contention by some that the practical requirements of their role do not require this.

References

Baty P 2006 Mark-up of 14% gave "fails" a pass. The Times, Higher Educational Supplement, April 21st, p. 7

Bleasdale A 1982 Boys from the black stuff. BBC, London

Butterworth P 1988 Breaking the boundaries. Council of Deans and Heads of UK University Nursing Faculties, Tavistock Square, London

Department of Health 2006 From values to action: the Chief Nursing Officer's review of mental health nursing. Department of Health, London

Johnston P 1998 Nursing crisis blamed on cultural failure. The Daily Telegraph, October 26th, p. 7

Lakeman R 1998 Beyond glass houses in the desert: a case for a mental health care system. Journal of Psychiatric and Mental Health Nursing 5(4):324–328

Le Var R 1997a Project 2000: a new preparation for practice – has policy been realized? Part 1. Nurse Education Today 17(3): 171–177

Le Var R 1997b Project 2000: a new preparation for practice – has policy been realized? Part 2. Nurse Education Today 17(4):263–273

Marrin M 1999 Nurses are the problem. The Sunday Telegraph, January 10th, p. 31

Martin E 1999 Nurses and higher education. Council of Deans and Heads of UK University Nursing Faculties, Tavistock Square, London

McKenzie R 2005 Am I flogging a dead metaphor? Sloppy scholarship and the implied spider. Journal of Psychiatric and Mental Health Nursing 12:550–555

Menzies-Lyth I 1988 Containing anxiety in institutions. Free Association Books, London

Murray I 1999 Back to the bedpans for student nurses. The Times, January 16th, p. 1

O'Reilly J 1999 University in £8m crisis faces break up. The Sunday Times, February 21st, p. 5

Phillips M 1999 How the college girls destroyed nursing. The Sunday Times, January 10th, p. 13

Radford J 1997 The changing purpose of higher education. In: Radford J, Raaheim K, deVries P et al (eds) Quantity and quality in higher education. Jessica Kingsley, London, pp. 7–47

Rosen P 2003 Education: dear Dianne Abbott. Socialist Review, December. Online. Available: http://www.socialistreview.org.uk

Tomey A M, Alligood M R 2006 Nursing theorists and their work. Elsevier Mosby, St. Louis, Missouri

Tomlinson M 2002 Inquiry into A Level standards: final report. Caxton House, London

Vere-Jones E 2006a Nursing come full circle. Nursing Times 102(9):16–17

Vere-Jones E 2006b Mental health manifesto. Nursing Times 102(17):14–17

Walden G 1996 We should know better: solving the educational crisis. Fourth Estate, London

While A 1999 Nursing shortages are not the fault of education. British Journal of Community Nursing 4(2):99

Williamson J 1998 Nursing grudges. The Daily Telegraph, March 1st, p. 32

Woodcock A 2006 Kelly confident over school reforms bill. The Independent, February 28th, p. 2

17

Role, responsibility and the structuring of mental health nursing students

You cannot get a quart into a pint pot

(*Daily News* 1896, July 24th, p. 4)

Isn't it amazing the number of people, for example counsellors and psychotherapists, who, professing expertise in human affairs, proceed as unrestrainedly as the rest of us towards nicotine addiction, marital breakdown and nervous exhaustion. You would think that profound reflection on the human condition might yield some mastery over its vicissitudes, but no. Too often, in too many walks of life, chasms appear between what, theoretically, ought to be the case and what, practically, isn't. Ponder if you will the following quotes from three dissatisfied student nurses:

> *"Nursing students do not feel valued and we are not paid enough. We know being a nurse is hard work but we want to have the time and money to let off steam."*
> *"We were all failed for academic reasons but those students were good nurses and they were committed to the profession."*
> *"Clinical placements can make you feel like just a pair of hands, no supervision, no guidance ... having no one to listen to you."*

These complaints (reported in the Nursing Times 2005) don't sound new or unique and so are not easily dismissed as anecdotal or as the product of noxious elements within the overall student body. What they represent are mismatches between what is and what ought to be the case. Take the question of lack of money: to what extent is this peculiar to student nurses? We could all do with more money, nothing unique about that to students. And yet, there are monetary questions of a vaguely philosophical nature that *are* unique to student nurses. For example, many students – certainly the ones I talk to – imbue their studentship with distinct occupational values. When asked if they would forsake their bursaries and undertake nursing as if it were English literature or geography – that is, acquire a large debt, as well as an education – they invariably say 'no'. They see the bursary as an intrinsic right but will often work extra hours, selling themselves through nursing agencies, so as to bolster it. Memory is a factor here and many nursing students know that, until it joined the universities, nurse education ran parallel to employee status; in effect, by the time you qualified, you were already three years into your pension. It may have been anticipated that the creation of Project 2000 would have killed this occupational mindset. However, imbued with a century of asylum/hospital trade unionism, as well as institutional shift systems that resemble industrial practice, it's a mindset that is deeply resistant to change. Indeed, so strong is this link that the anticipation of guaranteed employment upon qualifying remains unchanged.

NURSING CULTURE

My belief is that the bursary sustains the occupational attitude of nursing students as qualitatively different to other university students. In effect, nursing students are neither one thing nor another, their ambivalence confirmed by a bursary system which denotes employee status, a status made more explicit by frequent declarations that the money is 'never enough'. To an extent, these declarations were exacerbated by the *Making a Difference* reform (DoH 1999) of Project 2000 courses which had the effect of returning students to a working week in clinical practice but without an accompanying switch from bursary to salary. This particular change was partly driven by complaints about too much theory and insufficient preparatory clinical practice. However, one cannot be condemned for thinking, however cynically, that it constituted a ploy by which labour might be obtained on the cheap. Another point is that switching to a salaried status would have ruined the illusion of university student status.

One could, alternatively, argue that contemporary students receive a much more sophisticated and intensive supervision when on clinical placements than did their forebears, that they are not merely pairs of occupational hands, and many do assert this. Says lead nurse Suzi O'Connor:

> *"I think nurses are respected more as a profession now. Services are often ●nurse-led and we work as equals with other health*

professionals – we're not the crap ones in the team. We're no longer seen as the handmaidens."

(Vere-Jones 2006, p. 16)

We live, after all, in an era of quality assurance, awash with Quality and Assurance Agency and Nursing and Midwifery Council outcomes, objectives, formulae, proficiencies and criteria. Current practice is prescribed, its details set out in educational curricula so finely tuned in their constituent parts that even the medieval theologians, who debated the number of angels that could sit on a pinhead, would be put to shame. It hardly surprises that practice supervisors, faced with the task of translating these documents into practice, often respond antagonistically towards them as they do also to their constant re-jigging by educationalists (in search of the perfect curriculum). Students, too, are inundated with paper work, required to construct literary evidence that they have achieved this or that skill, mammoth documentation whose prevalence suggests a lack of trust or confidence in student mentors or, perhaps, a desire to hold them to account.

ORIGINAL CURRICULA

The original nursing syllabi were pared-down, enabling instruments distributed from London and enforced by occasional visits from General Nursing Council (GNC) and English National Board for Nursing, Midwifery and Health Visiting (ENB) inspectors/advisors. That these advisors confined themselves largely to the physical environment – 'the toilets seem dangerously close to the dining area' – or to teacher/student ratios or library resources suggests that there existed quite strong agreement about what constituted a decent nurse education. As the ENB superseded the GNC, matters became more academically complicated; still, nurse education remained grounded intellectually, and professionally, within schools still linked (geographically and organisationally) to practice. In fact, until the 1970s, nurse training schools were only nominally administered by tutors, being answerable ultimately to chief nursing officers. I recall a particular instance of this arrangement where my nurse training school had to battle for the transfer of students' files from service administration offices to the school itself.

I think that place is probably a factor here: current nursing students do not inhabit college campuses as though they belonged there and this contrasts strongly with the bonded experiences that were part and parcel of, and perhaps even constituted, the old nursing schools.

Comparing courses, past and present, nurse tutor Anthony Kinder (2005, p. 16) states: 'the older way was better in many respects' and that 'rampant MRSA or patients being left in corridors [or] dirty wards were unheard of'. While these particular points are contestable as outcomes of an inappropriate or inefficient education, what is nonetheless clear is that where mismatches develop between people and the organisations they serve, the problems that Kinder raises are precisely those most likely to occur. One would have thought, in an era of holistic practice, that disharmony would be minimal, that treatment centres would cohere around a central principle of comprehensive care and treatment. Yet, while contemporary students are taught holistic principles ad nauseam, they then enter practice settings wherein holism becomes secondary to professional boundary setting, fragmentation of identity or, at best, a division of labour in which responsibility becomes somebody else's problem. This may not involve an outright abrogation of responsibility; however, it does reflect nurses' attempts to corral knowledge and practice so as to exclude tasks no longer deemed appropriate to them.

IDENTITY AND RESPONSIBILITY

The social psychology literature (Myers 2004) comprehensively sets out how identity relates to responsibility. If you want people to work scrupulously, and carry out certain responsibilities, then it's no good ordering or even instructing them how to do it. You must inculcate (in them) a sense of their involvement, their ownership of the question at hand and its likely solutions. I believe that the old hospital training schools elicited from students a sense of being valued by virtue of instilling (in them) collegially defined aims. True, the nature of some of these values might be debatable but collegiality is important nevertheless and its absence corrodes accountability and the notion of norms of care.

I recall the vigorous trade union campaign that preceded the Halsbury (DHSS 1974a) restructuring of salaries and in particular the remarkable images of chief nursing officers visiting picket lines to provide some moral support. I am not suggesting that relationships within the nursing hierarchy were plain sailing: some managers' attitudes towards staff smacked of 'well, they may be fools but they're my fools', but this did reflect a certain benevolent camaraderie. It's a camaraderie and a benevolence that is long gone. Such cohesion, of course, was made possible by the autonomy that comes with power: until the 1980s nursing occupied a commanding position in NHS management possessing both fiscal power and the authority of knowledge. With the advent of Thatcherism, nurse administration was emasculated, becoming in the process a conduit for higher administrative forces and a new-found political consensus that professions needed to be controlled. For nurses, the fall from managerial grace was slow but uneventful, culminating in a roster of managers whose service was to corporate interests, and the notion that a nurse manager might visit a picket line today is risible.

Comparing this to the parallel progress of police constabularies reveals interesting differences between the two. Notice, for example, that when chief constables appear in public they are invariably in uniform, thus making visible links between themselves and other ranks. Following the reorganisation of nursing management (DHSS 1966) the first thing the new nursing officers did was throw off all semblance of uniform: they became the original men (and women) in suits. Although their job descriptions included clinical as well as administrative responsibilities, they quickly fell into an overly hierarchic managerialism in most cases embarking on graded executive style courses and assuming professional authority by means of promotion.

It's also worth contrasting – in the light of comparative complexities and lengths of training involved – how both police and nurses have fared with successive governments, especially in respect of pay structures and working conditions. Nursing would seem to have lost collective identity and so is constantly exposed to interpretation and definition by others, including governments. Yet again, for example, mental health nursing has been reviewed (Strachan-Bennett 2005), the orientation of its functions top of the agenda. Historians will have a field day working out the ambivalences behind the invention of 'consultant' nurses and the re-emergence of 'matron' occurring in the same epoch. It is worth comparing the divergent political impulses which drove these two developments: although both could be seen as equally redemptive for a profession perceived as failing – failing in its standards of hygiene, its lack of accountability – one was premised on a plane of expertise and professionalised knowledge while the other was seen as a means of accountability, rigour and the re-imposition of order. Whether one opts for one or other of these, or elements from both, their dual manifestation within the body politic suggests disarray within the profession overall.

OCCUPYING ORGANISATIONS AND THE RADICAL 1960S

One of the advantages of organisations with defined rules and goals is that their members come to know, intuitively, what works and what doesn't. In the past, what worked in the training schools was bolstered by agreements about what constituted the well-trained nurse. However, the encroaching radicalism of the times implicitly warned against closed systems and organisations which militated against personal liberty. Ervin Goffman (1968) trenchantly dissected the malevolent processes that entwined all organisations such that his – well-impressed – readers, fearing heresy, shied away from critiquing his work. But although intended as a critique of institutionalisation, Goffman's 'totality' – the extent to which institutions are impervious to outside influences – may be seen, retrospectively, untypically, as not all that pernicious. We have been led to believe that institutions fomented destructive forces and there is evidence for this (DHSS 1974b). The received wisdom supports the old mental hospitals as empires of regimentation inducing burnout in their inmates. At the same time, some view the asylums/hospitals as products of altruism and Victorian benevolence (Jones 1972), that they were the best option in the circumstances, that they created role, order and purpose for all those within them. Similarly, the ordering of general hospitals within communities, often with identifying names that fixed them in history, and with distinctive uniforms and closely defined – authoritarian perhaps – roles, also facilitated purpose, loyalty and the inculcation of high standards of hygiene and efficiency. Perceptions of role and responsibility relate closely to identity: today's students are required to work, uncomfortably, within frameworks of ambivalence. At times – look again at the second student quote above – they cannot even be confident that they are failing for the right reasons. Or look at this further example from a second-year student:

> *"I am being discontinued because of my poor academic writing style, even though I have passed exams and my clinical skills and I had brilliant reports from my mentor. Things have moved for the worse and the old system of learning where you did it all 'in house' is the way to train."*

(Brown 2004, p. 33)

Or this from a second-year student who is already a university graduate:

> *"Most people who want to be nurses are practical people and want to be trained for a career that celebrates that practicality and not their ability to wax lyrical on the theoretical underpinnings of the job."*

(Chearman 2006, p. 12)

Such academic fare is problematic to them (and their practice supervisors) because, by now, they have probably experienced success in the practice arena and what this entails. Indeed, failure in this arena is so rare that students must surely suppose that opposing forces are at play. This may intensify further when subject matter pushed by academics is seen as unduly abstract. The ambivalence extends everywhere; for example, observe how students are required to occupy classrooms for nigh on 25 hours a week, a predilection (of adult nurse lecturers) that not only connects to *what* is taught but, more so, to what *ought* to be taught and how. It's as if nursing schools, on joining the universities, are failing to acquire some of the basic precepts by which they work. Thus, the carry-over of extensive teacher-centred classroom sessions and the insistence that students attend everything, measured in many institutes by roll calls and/or attendance registers. This approach may be pertinent to adult nurses who must match a curriculum supposedly grounded in humanist principles with efficient practice in medical settings. I say supposedly because I suspect the problem is partly solved by a (hidden) agenda of medical information for which full attendance at lengthy classroom sessions is required. This is probably not a bad thing and adult students, certainly at pre-registration level, do not object to it. But the overall effect is of nursing institutes operating furtively, partially camouflaging nursing school agendas behind a veneer of higher education concerns. So that there takes place the usual round of meetings and seminars, espousing the jargon and maintaining the bureaucracy of college life but with splits between this and classroom practice. The double sidedness is necessary because it lessens the chasm between theory and practice by simply diminishing the theory. However, this brings with it more contradiction, for while many nurse teachers extol the virtues of 'practice-based learning', the third student quote at the start of this chapter suggests that this type of learning and its supervision are elusive. No doubt standards of supervision vary (Harrison 2006) and, for instance, special units (such as forensic psychiatry) will be more enabling because they are better staffed and/or funded. As a generalisation, however, embracing the university mantle has led to further widening of the practice–theory gap. Specifically, that gap has been concretised by the geographical distance between psychiatric students' clinical placements and the campuses to which they must travel for their theory. This cannot but inflate the psychological remoteness of theory from what they identify as necessary through practice and service mentorship. From this emerges their sense of division: it becomes difficult for them to develop a locus of control, purpose or structure.

WHAT IS TO BE TAUGHT?

If there is prior agreement about what is to be taught – in effect, what is important to nursing, what characterises its functions – then this should possess at least a scintilla of definition. In a wide-ranging attempt to bring definitions to nursing (RCN 2003, p. 1) one expert committee included the following:

> *"If we cannot name it, we cannot control it, finance it, research it, teach it or put it into public policy."*

A particular difficulty with this is that, traditionally, nurses have resolutely refused to examine their basic functions, what nursing is and what it isn't. This has been a complaint (of mine) for years, that we proceed as if basic issues of role and identity have been resolved when, over the years, matters have become more disjunctive and confused. Take, for instance, the question of cognitive behaviour therapy (CBT). Some nurses inhabit this role although a fair number of them drop the word nurse from their title when they do; others insist on the word nurse as a descriptor, jealously asserting their nursing identity. However, there is a problem with this assertion which is not that easy to resolve; perhaps the following dual scenario may provide some resolution.

Imagine you are passing two adjacent windows and that inside each is a patient – Mrs Jones or Mrs Smith – both of whom have a diagnosis of agoraphobia; both are of similar age, are from similar socio-economic backgrounds and have the same type and degree of disturbance. Behind one window Mrs Jones receives CBT from a psychiatric nurse; behind the other, Mrs Smith receives CBT from a clinical psychologist. My question is: 'What would you observe that would lead you to think that one practitioner was a nurse and one was not?' Whenever I pose this question, the typical audience response is that the nurse will display qualities (of caring) and the psychologist either won't or won't to the same extent. It is claimed that nurses possess humanitarian instincts that are somehow missing in other clinical therapy groups. Such arrogance – grounded in little more than personal reflection aided and abetted by a misplaced idealism – is hardly a careful working through of what psychiatric nursing is about; it lacks precision and so is easy to refute. In itself, the two-windows scenario doesn't diminish the place of humanistic instincts in nursing, but it does question the proprietorial claims of nurses that they are the exemplars of this, the sole heirs of Carl Rogers.

I would like to conclude this chapter by examining two attempts to define nursing: one that tries to do this on the basis of borrowed principles and another which views collaborative research as holding out the best promise of professional uniqueness. To do this I will draw from a book of essays (Tilley 2005) on states of nursing knowledge. In a well-argued chapter, Desmond Ryan (2005, p. 218) reflects that although the 'nurse–patient relationship is central to the discussion [of fields of nursing knowledge] practical knowledge bearing on that relationship rarely figures in [this] book'. When it does, he observes, the knowledge base in question – psychoanalysis – is of distinctly non-nursing origins. The issue, of course, is not just psychoanalysis: one could substitute any borrowed theory – cognitive behaviour theory or medical (psychiatric) practice – and the point still stands, which is that we are no nearer an *internally* derived theory of nursing than we have ever been. The problem for nursing theorists is to extricate themselves from social, spatial and professional contexts that are predefined by non-nursing discourses. This is what Foucault (1982) meant in his perorations on power, that it acquires leverage within localised areas, that because regionally constructed its business is mediated by circumscribed procedures, especially language. So, while nurses are now fully primed with humanistic theory, more expert at sociology than sociologists, this means that they always lack an articulation that does not sound as if borrowed from elsewhere. Although the failure of identity starts here, it is in practice, where the dominant language is medical, that final discontinuity of identity occurs. For example, the seeds of destruction of Project 2000 stemmed from its imposition from a centre that was either blithely unaware or simply ignorant of what usually passes as 'shop floor' nursing. Ryan (2005) puts it more elegantly: what you get left with in these circumstances, he says, are 'ideal types', what he calls 'abstractions which float free from any institutional linkage' (p. 219) or, in my view, which link into institutions in furtive ways. At this point, several conclusions follow and for clarity's sake, I will list them.

1. Nursing is a practice-based occupation which lacks a theory.
2. Adult nursing should acknowledge its debt to medical principles and accept its facilitative role in implementing these principles under medical direction.
3. Psychiatric nurses should seek to embrace one or other of the psychological, *not* psychiatric, theories so as to better inform and account for their practice.
4. Psychiatric nurses may, alternatively, embrace one of the humanistic approaches which may actually be necessary given the nature of some clients' problems.

It remains to say that if psychiatric nurses adopt either items 3 or 4 above then it becomes questionable to what extent they can still cling to a nursing identity, since both approaches are the property of other disciplines. They could, however, devise a language that makes a claim to precede item 4, nursing as the progenitor of person centredness. This would take them to a realm in which 'being with' and attending to non-medical needs would be their proper metier.

References

Brown J 2004 Letters section. Nursing Standard 18(45):33

Chearman J 2006 Listen up. Nursing Times 102(23):12

Department of Health 1999 Making a difference. HMSO, London

Department of Health and Social Security 1966 Report of the Committee on Senior Nurse Staffing Structure. HMSO, London

Department of Health and Social Security 1974a Report of the Committee of Inquiry into the Pay and Related Conditions of Nurses and Midwives. HMSO, London

Department of Health and Social Security 1974b Report of the Committee of Inquiry into South Ockendon Hospital. HMSO, London

Foucault M 1982 Afterword: the subject and power. In: Dreyfus H L, Rabinow P (eds) Michel Foucault: beyond structuralism and hermeneutics. Harvester, Brighton

Goffman E 1968 Asylums. Penguin, Harmondsworth

Harrison S 2006 March of the mentors. Nursing Standard 20(27): 14–15

Jones K 1972 A history of mental health services. Routledge, London

Kinder A 2005 Letters section. Nursing Times 101(9):16

Myers D G 2004 Exploring social psychology, 3rd edn. McGraw-Hill, London

Nursing Times 2005 Letters section. Nursing Times 101(9):17

Royal College of Nursing (RCN) 2003 Defining nursing. RCN, London

Ryan D 2005 Dance of knowledge: play of power: intellectual conflict as symptom of policy contradiction in the field of nursing knowledge. In: Tilley S (ed.) Psychiatric and mental health nursing: the field of knowledge. Blackwell, Oxford, pp. 216–234

Strachan-Bennett S 2005 Looking towards a changing future. Nursing Times 101(8):12–13

Tilley S (ed.) 2005 Psychiatric and mental health nursing: the field of knowledge. Blackwell, Oxford

Vere-Jones E 2006 Mental health manifesto. Nursing Times 102(17):14–17

Drugs, euphemisms and cyborgs

SECTION CONTENTS

18 You say you want a revolution

It is one thing to show someone that they are in error and another to put them in possession of truth

(John Locke 1632–1704)

If something is said often enough, then even if untrue, it becomes truth through repetition. So it was that Richard Gray (2001) trotted out the phrase 'revolutionary' when describing the introduction of phenothiazine drugs into Britain in the 1950s. A self-confessed 'scientist', Gray (2005) stands in the vanguard of advocating collaborative work with the medical profession particularly in the field of medication and the use of randomised controlled trials (RCTs). This collaborative element finds expression in nursing within a two-tiered objective of acquiring powers of 'nurse prescribing' and managing the so-called problem of patients' non-compliance, or concordance, with medication. Of course, this love affair with drugs is not new and one doesn't have to question pharmacological efficacy without noting how some, within the nursing profession, continue to overrate them compared to other approaches.

The phenothiazines, especially, were accorded 'magic bullet' status when first introduced; they quickly merited the title 'major tranquillisers' being trumpeted as 'first choice' in the treatment of psychosis. They retain their fans: Professor Gournay's (2003) paper, *Drug treatments for schizophrenia: why they offer the* only *hope for patients* (my emphasis), is indicative of the weight they still carry in psychiatric nursing circles. However, the advent of more benign 'atypical tranquillisers' has pushed supporters of phenothiazines to belatedly acknowledge their destructive side effects, perhaps recognising their not quite revolutionary status after all. Actually, the phrase 'side effects' presupposes much: Gray (2001, p. 38) observes that tardive dyskinesia, an especially troubling effect of anti-psychotics:

> *"can be particularly debilitating and once it has developed it is almost impossible to treat effectively."*

In fact, it is not reversible at all and, allowing its iatrogenic nature, it becomes a misnomer to call it a 'side effect' in any sense. Euphemisms like 'side effects' depreciate the ruinous effects of drugs, effects that attend a wide range of pharmacological treatments, psychiatric and non-psychiatric alike.

That said, in other areas of medicine benefits may outweigh deficits. Within psychiatry it can be asked if this is equally true; whether, for example, substituting a patient's delusional thinking with a drug-induced, irrevocable Parkinsonism is ethically fair exchange. The following extract (Gray 1998, p. 28–29) is of a patient trying to offset the imposition of compulsory medication: in it, 'J' tries to explain to his consultant 'C' what happens when he takes his antipsychotic medication.

J: I'm not coming here OK to be given drugs that I don't need, yeah to be injected in my private parts, kept under files. I came out of this hospital hardly able to brush my teeth, hardly able to eat, hardly able to stand. Now, what sort of medicine is that?

C: (attempting to interject) Can I ask you?

J: H h hold on. You keep me here by force. Wh wh what sort of, um, medical practition is that?

C: (attempting to interrupt) Let me take it one by one OK? You've been admitted under Section Two. It's a compulsory order: it means you have to stay in hospital …

J: You answer my question, that's what I want

C: I I'm doing that, all right. Now, it's up to four weeks …

J: No, no, no, no. Listen, listen, listen: if I came under your treatment am I supposed to leave better or worse?

C: I hope you leave much better.

J: It's not I hope. Um it's talking about what you did in the past. Yes?

C: I don't know about the past

J: You don't know? Listen, listen, you don't know about the past?

Examining this excerpt, Gray (1998) perceives the consultant as unwilling to engage in 'reciprocity' or 'dialogue' – although J does manage to interject some of his biography into the discussion. Gray quotes Laing (1990, p. 92) who says that:

> *"The role of patient tends to become defined as a non-agent, as a non-responsible object, to be treated accordingly."*

Critical to this objectification is the forcible administration of drugs via a set of formalities – J's legal status and a somewhat vaguely expressed diagnosis. His consultant describes the latter thus:

"Schizophrenia is a complex disorder which is characterized by strange bizarre beliefs which we call delusions – strange experiences, called hallucinations – hearing voices talking about you. He's never talked about hearing voices and he's never given evidence of what's called thought disorder, but I've no doubt that this is a schizophrenic illness."

(Gray 1998, p. 31)

On such contradictory grounds does much of contemporary psychiatric practice rest. This is not to say that we abandon psychiatric medicine but that we critically evaluate the part nurses play in its forcible administration, that we take account of patients' feelings and thoughts, that we do not arbitrarily medicate without considering legal, medical and ethical nostrums from everyone's perspective.

REVOLUTIONS

The 'revolutionary' tag awarded the phenothiazines reflected a determination by doctors such as William Sargant (1967) – in his day the foremost physical treatment psychiatrist in Britain – to medicalise psychiatric practice. Sargant was thrilled about physical treatments, especially 'wonder drugs', and interminably asserted their capacity to conquer mental illnesses altogether. When, at the same time, social changes began to influence hospital practices, for example the open door movement of the 1950s (Clarke 2004), medicalists quickly linked such changes, including an embryonic community psychiatric service, to the new drugs. In effect, they mistook correlation for cause and effect and, eager to fill the conceptual gap between open doors and their positive effects, manufactured a causative model whereby change was ascribed to the drugs.

Explaining changes in British hospital psychiatry in the 1950s is not straightforward. Certainly, the phenothiazines helped calm some behaviours of anti-social and suicidal patients and were a useful adjunct to progressive change. However, as I have shown (Clarke 2004), the doors of many British hospitals were open *before* these drugs were widely prescribed. Dingleton Hospital, Scotland, for instance, had all of its doors open, inside and out, by 1948. However, a linear, pharmacological, cause–effect explanation proved attractive, perhaps unsurprisingly, given the comparative difficulty of locating patients' wellbeing within family, economic and social systems. With benefit of hindsight, however, some socio-analytical psychiatrists (Clark 1991, Jones 1982) established important implications drawn from their 1939–1945 war experiences and its aftermath.

Specifically, they had observed seemingly well soldiers going to war but returning from 'the front' in need of psychiatric help. Two conclusions were drawn from this: first, the idea of mental illness as 'inborn and irredeemable', as a product of brain dysfunction and/or heredity, was dealt a hammer blow. Second, this discovery stimulated developments in social psychiatry, most notably the emergence of therapeutic communities. These were of two types: the socio-rehabilitative communities pioneered by Maxwell Jones (1982) at the Henderson Hospital, and the psychoanalytic approach championed by Tom Main (1989) and Wilfred Bion (1961) primarily at the Tavistock Clinic.

Although these progressions enabled a social construction model of mental breakdown to emerge, this did not replace the dominant emphasis on individual pathology and, apart from some major centres of innovation, filtering social constructionist thinking into more than small numbers of the major mental hospitals remained difficult. However, a theoretical social psychiatry became possible and institutions, such as the Tavistock, allowed for the continued study of mental distress particularly through the study of groups. At the same time, the high visibility of social psychiatrists and a growing radicalism made it *appear* that social constructionism was more prevalent than it was. This conjured the misperception that radical psychiatry had upended conventional practice, resulting in forms of psychiatric nurse training driven by post-1960s radical lecturers eager to belittle the achievements of medical science. The contemporary dominance of biological determinism speaks for itself, however, as does the current predilection of nursing's governing bodies for 'basic skills', the latter directed at meeting service-driven demands for better student acquaintance with drugs and other practical elements.

SEQUESTERING

Sequestering past events in support of contemporary agendas is an important part of acquiring control. In respect of psychiatry, asserting a theoretical base, supposedly arrived at by inexorable scientific advance, is about maintaining professional hegemony. Scientific psychiatry insists that it sits 'outside' society, adjudicating human behaviour, but is itself implicated in shaping society's norms to begin with. Philosopher Anthony Quinton (1985, p. 32) refers to:

> *"the tight lipped evasiveness of psychiatric professionalism [where] disease is defined in purely statistical terms."*

What he means is that psychiatrists define mental illness as abnormal outcomes of biology but with abnormality determined statistically, in the sense of setting it against yardsticks of 'normality'. This provides psychiatry with a scientific assuredness by which to define behaviours as abnormal but without examining why. Quinton notes how humans share much physicality in common – for example, temperature and skeletal structure – statistical variations of which can lead to diagnosis. Mentally, however, we differ more widely with huge amounts of historical, environmental, psychological and religious factors, precisely the factors which bring in evaluative elements when deciding about the presence or absence of mental health, and this is where the difficulties lie. For if we force detention and treatment on someone because they are a danger to themselves or others, by what criteria do we leave heavy cigarette smokers alone? It has to be because of the quality of mind behind why individuals do things and not what they actually do. Yet, paradoxically, it is what they do that gets people diagnosed, sectioned, detained and/or forcibly treated. And if one challenges this on grounds that many patients are voluntary, then, as Larry Gostin (1977) retorts, how do we know what transpires between professionals and demoralised patients in their front parlours as they are *persuaded* to consent to treatment? Are we so naïve that we believe that differences between voluntary and detained status in psychiatry are absolute?

THE MADNESS STATE

The concept of what qualifies as 'the madness state' is left open because psychiatrists are trained to act on symptoms, as are psychiatric nurses. Only one psychiatrist, Thomas Szasz (1997), has addressed this issue, albeit so stridently as to make his arguments seem ill-judged. His position proceeds along two fronts: to begin with, he states that because mental illness lacks a physical basis – a visible pathology – then it cannot be illness. For example, it cannot compare to heart disease where anatomical changes are measured against the relative severity of patients' symptoms. Second, he says that mental illnesses are just forms of behaviour – difficult to contend with, yes, but not to be construed as illness. To do so removes from affected individuals rights they would otherwise retain in law. Szasz has been influential and he is quoted endlessly although, one suspects, by those with both a literal view of things and an inability to see that his polemic is more about anger than logic. He is, in fact, wrong in the first part of his 'argument': many illnesses do not have detectable pathological bases so mental illness is not alone here.

When, in 1854, Dr John Snow removed the handle from the Broad Street pump, deaths from cholera plummeted, despite the fact that the mechanism of the disease was unknown to anyone including Snow. James Parkinson described the illness which bears his name on clinical grounds and with no understanding of its underlying mechanisms. Similarly, today, much of back pain stems from inferred causes, and phenomena such as chest pain of unknown origin remain a mystery but no less real to sufferers for all that.

However, Szasz is right about behaviour: his contention that mental illnesses are really 'problems in living'. Having witnessed hundreds of hospitalised psychiatric patients I cannot recall a single one who was not annoying someone, somewhere, and where this was not an important factor in their detention. At a time of growing biological psychiatry Szasz continues his campaign against disempowerment of mentally ill people, sticking to his guns despite rising tides of rejection and ridicule. For example, consultant psychiatrist Dr Duncan Double, following scepticism about his non-organic approach to patients, was suspended under advice that he retrain in 'organic psychiatry'. His use of a website to publicise his views also did not help:

> *"Basically I was regarded as different. I was using less medication than many psychiatrists and was not so concerned about arriving at diagnoses."*

(James 2006, p. 21)

Although now holding a senior position within the NHS, Double doesn't doubt that his clinical position is still insecure since his work can be perceived as a threat to what he refers to as the 'bio-medical hegemony gripping contemporary psychiatric practice'.

Indeed, it is quite common for psychiatric critics to be maligned as idiosyncratic (see Scull 1993, p. 3) or out of touch. The radical psychiatrist R. D. Laing was highly conscious of how his work was received:

> *"You think I've cut into the conscience of everyone that Martin Roth teaches? My work has not made the slightest difference – in fact, it's only entrenched them."*

(Mullan 1995, p. 378)

Laing believed that medical psychiatrists, like Roth, had scant regard for ideas that differed from assumptions about the biology of mental distress; in many ways, Laing's work became a wake-up call for medicalists to garner yet *more* data in support of the biological view.

The ridicule persists and, today, critics of conventional psychiatry are derided as holed up in the past, unable to see the 'giant strides' that scientific psychiatry continues to make. Further, there is perpetrated the myth that Laing and others carried the day in the 1960s and after, and that their message was even more radical than it really was. According to Dalrymple (2005) anti-psychiatry preached that the hospitalisation of schizophrenics was dehumanising not only in its institutionalised procedures but more so because responsibility for the schizophrenic 'condition really lay with twisted, insightless, parents unapprised of the machinations of capitalist systems'. There is a smidgen of truth in this but it is an overstatement that anti-psychiatry:

"became extremely popular in an era that uncritically criticised all institutions [and that] these ideas paved the way for an ill-conceived and hasty deinstitutionalisation of the mentally ill."

(Dalrymple 2005, p. 112)

Deinstitutionalisation had earlier antecedents than this (Clarke 2004). Martin (1955) had introduced the concept of 'institutionalisation' as a critical exercise and this was quickly followed by Russell Barton's *Institutional Neurosis* (1957) which itemised how the social rules of hospitals induced clinical syndromes almost identical to chronic schizophrenia. In a seminal paper, Rees (1957) identified the 'Moral Treatment' of the 18th century as the genesis of psychiatric liberalism, the true beginnings of the social approach to treatment and rehabilitation. The upsurge of 1960s radical psychiatry had a stylish self-consciousness which made conventional psychiatry seem drab and pedantic. It had that 1960s verve which made it seem at the time – and for some still does – that the very foundations of society were unhinged. However, the seeds of change were much older and more modest in their aims and the revitalisation of medicalisation from about the early 1980s onwards is testimony to that.

PERSISTENCE

A remarkable aspect of nurses writing about drugs (see Bennett 1998) today is the denial of context, of sociality, culture or history: an unsurprising view in the case of biochemists, pharmacologists and medicalists, but nurses? One would expect nurses to go beyond pharmacological and biomedical descriptions and address some of the cultural factors that impact on patients' general welfare. Also, what kind of an objectivity eulogises the benefits of psychiatric drugs without noticing drug company profits or the lengths to which these companies go in pressuring medics into prescribing their products? Or, why do supporters of nurse prescribing ignore the scandal of medics being paid by drug companies to publish favourable reviews of their products in pharmacology and medical journals? Drugs are 'big business' and while, understandably, biochemists endorse their treatment properties, psychiatric nurses might reasonably be expected to address the issue of many patients *having* to take them, weighing their benefits against other investments in care. Positioning psychiatric nursing within a biomedical-pharmacological complex sidesteps critical faculties whose intellectual and emotional acuity arrive from different traditions. Those traditions imbue nurses with scepticism about psychiatric claims to scientific credibility; they facilitate a 'non-clinical' stance by which treating forcibly can be assessed against other factors. True, psychiatric service users may resist such approaches as professional condescension, insisting on speaking for themselves. For the moment, however, psychiatric nurses who call for collaboration with (and imitation of) psychiatric medicine risk losing sight of the ethnic, gender, economic and empowerment aspects of patients' lives.

THE UNHEALTHY PAST

Henry Ford said that 'history is bunk' and, remarkably, some psychiatric nurses also define concern with the past as unhealthy, especially when focusing on cultural or philosophical issues; the radical psychiatry of the 1960s, for example, is rejected as rhetoric and of little utility. Simultaneously, these nurses hail developments in diagnostics and physical treatments as 'ground breaking', psychiatry's only hope of defeating mental disorder, and they have become adept at finding a past that supports this. History thus becomes a battleground with different sides seeking legitimation for their respective positions. However, contemporary orthodoxies weaken when shown to rest on false assumptions. My generation was sold a psychiatric 'drug revolution' via a training system (of the 1970s) content to acquiesce to 'superior' medical wisdom. The anti-psychotic phenothiazines became a marker for medical achievement, the cornerstone by which psychiatrists emerged as 'first among equals'. It was even believed that anti-psychotics had mandated passage of the 1959 Mental Health Act when, in fact, this act had been in several pipelines for years and was hardly a consequence of new drugs. Its germinal status was the World Health Organisation's influential 3rd Report (1953) written by, among others, Dr Percival

Rees of Warlingham Park Hospital, an English pioneer of open door hospitals and community psychiatry.

A PSYCHOSOCIAL NURSING?

Yet, a radicalised, psychosocial nursing would quickly come unstuck. Like it or not, nursing is linked to medicine and redefining it as a qualitatively different activity remains problematic. The idea is not new: the Peggy Jay Committee (Jay 1979) recommended the abolition of mental handicap nursing – as it was then called – and its replacement by carers trained in social work. The committee's proposals, vehemently rejected by the nurses, were shelved but their effect accelerated change, and learning disability nurses quickly demedicalised their roles but, in the process, became unrecognisable as nurses. To an extent, the abolitionist stance of the Jay Committee was feasible because, for most learning disabled people, the nature of the problem is one of learning and not illness.

For psychiatric nurses to break with psychiatry, alternatively, would involve them casting aside beliefs about mental illness and this is unlikely. And yet, psychiatric nurses *have* tried to represent themselves to patients in ways that medical practice disallows. For example, they have argued the importance of re-centring patients as 'persons', working from standpoints that attend closely to patients' experiences (Barker & Buchanan-Barker 2005). This was the sense in which Anthony Clare remarked how, in the 1960s, R. D. Laing had 'put the person back into the patient' as indeed he had. It has always been my belief that Laing was the perfect psychiatric nurse as his early work in the back wards of Glasgow's Gartnavel Hospital shows. His first paper was published in a nursing journal and he had that extraordinary affinity with psychotic people which comes from tacit understanding rather than formal theory. As Coppock & Hopton (2000, p. 72) recall, Laing believed that meaningful communication with psychotic people was the essence of care, whereas they observe that at the time:

> *"clinical descriptions of schizophrenia in most psychiatric textbooks often resembled characterisations in gothic horror films."*

The following is typical of a 1960s description:

> *"Delusions of a bizarre or fantastic nature occur and such patients frequently show a silly fatuous manner, their behaviours being foolish, erratic and accompanied by mannerism and strange antics."*

(Ackner 1964, p. 146)

Compare this with Gray's (2001, p. 38) description of the same group:

> *"The condition is characterised by a range of symptoms, the most common being hallucinations, delusions, thought disorder, impaired cognitive functioning, social isolation and lack of motivation."*

While differences attend both these descriptions, the general tenor of the latter is clinical and sanitised of social and cultural influences. Yet, what to replace the clinical perspective with? If these 'person-centred' approaches are to be believed, then nothing – or very little – is needed over and above a *relationship* (with patients). Others, however, see this as insufficient to deal with all but the most 'minor' psychological difficulties and that something like schizophrenia requires a response over and above what is given in relationships or friendship. Discussing this, psychiatrists Pat Bracken and Phil Thomas (2004, p. 10), who work with a full complement of patients, stated:

> *"Since its origins in the European Enlightenment, psychiatry has been anxious to proclaim that its treatments are based on scientific research, and has played down the importance of such things as faith, hope and the importance of values and meanings."*

Bracken & Thomas practise what they call 'post-psychiatry' which seems to play down scientistic thinking so as to recover a practical psychiatry based on hope and 'relationship building'. Their final exposition (2004, p. 10):

> *"is that the most important things that have shaped our lives have been the stories, lives and experiences of people (friends, colleagues and patients) who have gone through episodes of madness and distress. Post-psychiatry, if it stands for nothing else, stands in tribute to their courage, suffering, humour and strength."*

This, however, still begs the question of what one brings to suffering over and above love, friendship and concern. Few would deny that pharmacological efficacy is enhanced when drugs are administered in a warm and life-enhancing way and we know that psychotic people react more positively in forgiving and non-judgemental contexts (Leff 1984). So that even if one's orientation is clinical, this doesn't mean tossing aside the ordinary decencies of everyday life. But it is stretching things to suggest that 'all you need is love' if people are psychotic or if gripped by obsessive compulsions. In these cases, in addition to hope and courage, psychological interventions of established merit are needed.

MOVING ON

Pitting assertions against each other without sight of agreement or resolution is circular and tedious. At the same time, trying to distinguish between compliance and coercion continues to divide psychiatric nurses as does the relative place of patients' narratives within the recovery process. Because many psychotic people are helped by drugs, nurses should of course know their effects (both desired and undesired). However, the nursing role is to operate between the patients' medical status and his or her life. This role is not intrinsic to the physiological effects of medication: rather does it approach issues of medication from broader perspectives. That many psychiatric nurses persist in centralising medication is but a continuation of that process that began with the 'revolutionary' standing accorded these drugs in the 1950s. We need not be surprised, when medication is refused, that patients are designated 'non-compliant' as though this was integral to their mental state, as though it could never be a straightforward refusal by someone who feels threatened. No doubt, a concept of 'psychiatric refusenik' will one day win some recognition; until then we will continue to designate patients as objects to which we are subject. We will continue to describe iatrogenic disease – tardive dyskinesia – as a 'side effect' thus softening the untoward consequences of 'treatments'. There has to be more to psychiatric nursing than abject acquiescence to an orthodoxy that allows drug companies to list what the 'side effects' are and so make their products more user friendly. Addressing these questions does not mean abandoning ideas of psychiatric disorder or its treatment; it puts pressure on such concepts, however, and it shunts psychiatric nurses towards a less controlled (and controlling) practice.

References

Ackner B 1964 Handbook for psychiatric nurses. Baillière Tindall, London

Barker P, Buchanan-Barker P 2005 The tidal model: a guide for mental health professionals. Brunner-Routledge, Hove

Barton R 1957 Institutional neurosis. John Wright, Bristol

Bennett J 1998 Antipsychotic drug treatment. Mental Health Practice 1(5):29–34

Bion W 1961 Experiences in groups and other papers. Tavistock, London

Bracken P, Thomas P 2004 Hope. Openmind 130:10

Clark D H 1991 Maxwell Jones and the mental hospitals. International Journal of Therapeutic Communities 7:117–123

Clarke L 2004 The time of the therapeutic communities. Jessica Kingsley, London

Coppock V, Hopton J 2000 Critical perspectives on mental health. Routledge, London

Dalrymple T 2005 In the asylum. City Journal 15(3):108–116

Gostin L 1977 A human condition. MIND, London

Gournay K 2003 Drug treatments for schizophrenia: why they offer the only hope for patients. Mental Health Practice 6(6):16–17

Gray B T 1998 The politics of psychiatry and community care: a discourse analytic approach to the case study of John Baptist. Changes 16(1):24–37

Gray R 2001 Medication for schizophrenia. Nursing Times 97(31): 38–39

Gray R 2005 A framework for development and evaluation of RCTs for complex interventions to improve health. Paper given at the 11th International NPNR Conference at Oxford University, September 28th

James A 2006 My tutor said to me, this talk is dangerous. The Times, Higher Education Supplement, April 21st, p. 21

Jay P 1979 Report of the Committee of Inquiry into Mental Handicap Nursing and Care. HMSO, London

Jones M 1982 The process of change. Routledge, London

Laing R D 1990 The politics of experience and the bird of paradise. Penguin, London

Leff J 1984 Expressed emotion in families: its significance for mental illness. Guilford Press, New York

Main T 1989 The ailment and other psychoanalytic essays. Free Association Books, London

Martin D 1955 Institutionalization. Lancet, 3rd December, 1188–1190

Mullan B 1995 Mad to be normal: conversations with R D Laing. Free Association Books, London

Quinton A 1985 Madness. In: Phillips Griffiths A (ed.) Philosophy and practice. Cambridge University Press, Cambridge, pp. 17–41

Rees T P 1957 The unlocked door. Lancet, November 6th, 953–954

Sargant W 1967 The unquiet mind. Heienmann, London

Scull A 1993 The most solitary of afflictions: madness and society in Britain 1700–1900. Yale University Press, London

Szasz T 1997 The manufacture of madness. Syracuse University Press, New York

World Health Organisation 1953 Expert Committee on Mental Health 3rd Report. WHO, Geneva

19

Euphemistically challenged

Fine words butter no parsnips

(Clarke 1639)

During the 1960s it became public knowledge that the US Government was putting a chemical substance into its water supply: that substance, fluoride, announced US officials, would protect the nation's teeth from decay. In Stanley Kubrick's (1964) film *Dr Strangelove or: How I Learned to Stop Worrying and Love the Bomb*, a psychotic general, Jack D. Ripper, believes that fluoridating water is a communist conspiracy aimed at polluting the nation's bodily fluids, the result being 'loss of essence' and an inability to procreate. Somehow, the general associates the 'putrefaction' of drinking water with the ebbing of his own bodily fluids and projects this onto the nation at large. Responding to the conspiracy, he orders American air force planes to launch a nuclear attack on Russia. When challenged as to why, Ripper acknowledges his belief in the fluoride conspiracy but remains coy about why it bothers him:

> *"And I can swear to you, my boy, swear to you, that there's nothing wrong with my bodily fluids, not a thing. I do not avoid women, Mandrake, but I do deny them my essence."*

The encounter classically demonstrates subterfuge and euphemism – a mad general executing verbal detours around his *impotence* by linking it to aquatic putrefaction – while displacing his rage on to the Russians who (who else?) become the real culprits.

POLITICIANS

While the late politician Alan Clark had been, as he put it, 'economical with "the actualite" ', some pundits took the view that he had lied. Clark's diary (1993) regaled readers with intriguing concoctions of fact and fiction that he was given to calling a 'work of art': art, after all, excuses everything. But, probably no contemporary politician has shown such adeptness at 'truthfully telling lies' as William Jefferson Clinton. Although he categorically declared 'I have not had sexual relations' with Ms Lewinski, several court judges and the US House of Representatives, which impeached him, begged to differ. What Clinton craftily concealed was that he had not had sexual *intercourse* with Ms Lewinsky, which, it seems, he hadn't. Everything hangs, you see, on what is meant by 'sexual relations'. In fact, the equivocation became his opt-out clause. If found out, he could simply affirm that what he had meant was that they had not had sexual intercourse. In fairness to Bill, the Concise Oxford English Dictionary (1977) defines 'sexual intercourse' as 'sex act': unfortunately, it doesn't specify which orifices may be involved.

NOT WHAT BUT HOW

In most endeavours these days, but especially in professional life, success is often a question of 'It ain't what you do, it's the way that you do it' or, more likely, the way that you are seen to do it. Today, the social audience is all: we are an age of packaging, sound bites, PR and spin-doctoring. Indeed, as much as how you do it, what may count even more is how you say you do it. Much of this has passed into health care: for example, the way in which nursing students are encouraged to build up portfolios which transform their studentship into something special. Hardly a study day or half-day conference goes by without it being certificated or credit rated. In respect of clinical work, recently a patient was informed that she was not, in fact, ill but that her broken leg (on traction) was 'a temporary and involuntary immobility contingent upon environmental assault' (by a lorry, incidentally). And as I write this, Secretary of State for Health, Patricia Hewitt, has just informed the Royal College of Nursing's Annual Conference, hours after being told that 13 000 jobs are potentially at risk, that the NHS has had its 'best year ever'.

In terms of our social and occupational lives, there are nowadays no sackings or redundancies, only downsizings; no cutbacks or shortages, only rationalisations; no 'control and restraint', only 'care and responsibility' (see Ch. 6); no psychiatry that is not mental health; no 'problems' that are not 'challenges and opportunities'. This last item set me on the linguistic trail of 'challenging behaviour' as a new and different category of human activity. The drive to establish secure psychiatric units within which 'challenging behaviour' would be contained intrigued me. Clearly, this was psychiatry at 'the cutting edge', a decisive response to a phenomenon that appeared (around the mid-1970s) to have come from nowhere in the way that psychological concepts – stress, normalisation, attention deficit disorder – tend to do.

BUT WHAT IS IT?

But exactly what is challenging behaviour? And, to whom is it challenging? As Gates (1997, p. 136) says:

> *"The use of the term is particularly problematic because it means different things to different people."*

In my dealings with patients, I had always found plaintiveness difficult to cope with; relentless laments of self pity and cravings for personal reassurance were beyond my capacity to serially satisfy. As a student, one was encouraged to behave towards patients in particular ways: it was important, for example, to be non-judgemental, to listen, to be empathic. The difficulty of being something you are not and what this means was never broached. I mean, how do you *be* empathic? For me, the struggle to *be* was precisely that, a struggle, and I often had to misrepresent myself to patients so as a) not to be unpleasant, b) to make the time pass while c) hoping that they would not see my pretence and d) on tenterhooks that if they did, they would at least thank me for trying. In any event, I had come to believe that understanding is an intolerable quality when not subject to critical revision; after all, what could be more wearying than the company of someone who understood you all the time? And besides, why should having a mental illness exempt anyone from the ordinary rules of social engagement? I found it easy to judge some patients for what I believed were normative transgressions even when other professionals thought this unwise and/or unethical. For my part, I believed the opposite: that what was ethical was to relate to patients as honestly as I could.

DIFFERENT STROKES

The fact is, that which you find challenging, I might find challenging for different reasons or not challenging at all. For example, a former patient of mine (with a severe learning disability) openly masturbated so frequently that his 'challenging behaviour' was countered with dollops of injected oestrogen, his enlarged breasts presumably being seen as less challenging. It is little comfort that such chemical violence would be frowned upon today, yet that, of course, is the point; that what challenges today may be innocuous tomorrow or, at least, deserving of different consideration.

In general, I suspect that 'challenging behaviour' denotes aggression, ranging from verbal abuse to violence, possibly self-inflicted, but often directed at professionals (Rose & Walker 1997). However, the term hardly signifies everything that challenges professionals since that would render it meaningless. Yet, that appears to be the case with the term only vaguely defined or not defined at all. In the past, difficult behaviour was managed in a variety of ways but, ultimately, by removing patients to 'refractory wards': refractory in the sense of sullen, disobedient, perverse, intransigent. Now, challenging behaviour has led to the construction of special units of segregation, modern equivalents of refractory wards, repositories for patients designated as malevolent, perhaps not violent but difficult to contain.

In many ways, secluding (or drugging) patients is a form of self-medication aimed at diminishing staff anxiety; secluding patients may also operate as a displacement of aggression towards them. Little has been written about how unconscious anxiety turns to apprehension about incipient 'patient aggression' and the creation of climates of violence wherein disturbances become all the more likely. Classically, challenging behaviours are seen as a product of the personality traits of patients coupled with environmental stresses of one kind or another. Professionals enter patients' worlds believing themselves to be objective arbiters of what they survey but they invariably fail to see how their subjective biases affect patients, setting up complexes of action–reaction where the origin of aggression, if it occurs, becomes difficult to pinpoint. Because challenging behaviour units are locked systems, this legitimises the custodial element of the nurses' role; this is ironic given that the history of psychiatric nursing is premised on a maturation from custodial to liberal/humanist positions. There is further irony in that contemporary forensic nursing is asserted to be more sophisticated, operating along lines of team work, better rationales and interdisciplinary strategies. However, heightened efficiency belies diminished reflectiveness leading to automated responding to patients' behaviours. During the hospital/asylum years, secluding patients was not as efficient as today but probably the more humane for all that. The old refractory wards nestled comfortably within the loose security of their hospital boundaries; modern units, purpose built and self reliant, have evolved in edgy isolation, nervously measuring their performance outcomes in security terms. These units always feel claustrophobic, their limited physical space rendering their inhabitants 'cabined, cribbed, confined' and potentially angry. In the past, refractory ward nurses accepted the 'reality' of nursing patients in locked and semi-locked systems. Aware that a critique of custodialism was brewing around them, they knew that developments like the 'open door movement' signalled the end of jangling keys and lockups. How surprised they must be, a generation later, seeing custodialism celebrated as an innovative response to a 'newly discovered' problem.

EVALUATING ACTIONS

Actually, until fairly recently psychiatric nurses hardly needed to consider the effects of their actions on patients: as an asylum/hospital nurse, punitiveness towards patients flowed from perceptions of them as suffering from irredeemable mental defects and so being ineligible for civil rights. Both nurses and their charges became caught up in institutionalised systems whose rules took on a life force of their own so that even mild reforms were seen as threatening. By the 1970s, however, a plethora of therapeutic models was bearing down on nursing practice: for example, behaviourist 'token economy' units were coming on stream, initially aimed at rehabilitating the anti-social behaviours of long-stay patients. One outcome of this activity was that the nursing vocabulary became more elaborate, aided and abetted by an expanding, more critically aware, educational curriculum. The field of learning disabilities, for instance, quickly absorbed behaviourist jargon and, very quickly, complex, exalted entries began appearing in patients' case notes. Fuelled by growing self-importance, nurses now declared that patients 'had failed to achieve optimum social potential' or that they 'were deficient in manual dexterity' or that they were exhibiting echopraxia, echolalia and so on. Such did this double speak flourish that it provoked New Zealand psychiatrist, Albert Kushlick (1996), to demand the return of concrete, descriptive terms when notating patients' behaviours. A much abused shorthand was the habit of describing epileptic fits as grand or petit mal seizures until someone pointed out that what mattered was less a French nomenclature and more the duration of unconsciousness, direction of fall, degrees of muscular contraction and so on: in other words, plain speaking and less of what Kushlick called 'fuzzies'.

ONE TOO MANY

Of current 'fuzzies' there is 'none more egregious than the vocabulary of challenging behaviour' (Mount 1997). It is hard to pinpoint when the term blossomed; probably around the late 1970s. At times of crisis and uncertainty it is not surprising that professionals seek to claim ancient territories or muster new ones in furtherance of their authority. Thatcherism ushered in a high nervousness for 'the professions', the hegemonic domains that had been theirs for years being called into question. There resulted a desperation to articulate positions of ascendancy, a striving for terminology that would make it *sound* as if some intractable or previously undefined problem had been solved or was at least being tackled. Phenomena such as attention deficit disorder (ADD) or repressed memory therapy (RMT) made their appearance, the latter intended to elicit childhood 'memories' of abuse as *the* harbinger of psychiatric disorder. That little evidence supported this hardly deterred practitioners of RMT. One ought to mention, also, the growing use this side of the Atlantic of the *Diagnostic and Statistical Manual of Diagnoses* (DSM-IV), a document whose shallowness derives from an extraordinary facility to proscribe everything but the kitchen sink as types of mental illness. R. D. Laing (Mullan 1999, p. 184) had scorned the DSM-IV arguing that:

> *"its excessively inclusive nature would be to culture out all manner of ordinary manifestations of ordinary minds, and that when all speech and conduct had been corrected we would be no more than homogenised creatures that we could barely recognize as human."*

For Harvard University psychiatrist Joseph Glenmullen (2005) the DSM-IV is nothing less than:

> *"a compendium of ... cursory, superficial menus of symptoms. Any attempt at helping patients understand themselves and to effect real change is lost in the rush to diagnose and medicate them."*

In addition to clinical psychiatry, the DSM-IV also stokes the ambitions of those involved in court custody cases, in education, indeed in any situation where mental illness, supposed or real, is a factor. The following are some of its recent additions: expressive language disorder, phonological disorder, sibling rivalry disorder, phase of life problem disorder, excessive gambling disorder, tobacco withdrawal disorder.

KIDS

In respect of children and adolescents, Mitchell (2003, p. 281) indicts the DSM-IV with:

> *"determining diagnoses such as conduct disorder or attention deficit hyperactivity disorder without sufficient critical regard for [their] ideological and historically situated assumptions."*

He goes on to say that the bald determinism of the DSM-IV concerning child development is profoundly restrictive and that a broader, rights-based approach would better account for children and young people's psychological distress. On a more commonplace, but equally serious, level the galloping autonomy of different disciplines has fragmented interventions designed to combat childhood abuse. What is needed are less discrete models of medical diagnosis and more an appreciation of the socio-political (especially family) backgrounds of childhood distress and trauma. We live in an increasingly disconnected world where 'the buck always stops elsewhere' and where accountability is difficult to nail down. The war against childhood abuse is a 'phoney war' (Mount 1997) that relies more on exclamations of disapproval, even horror, and less on forming an amalgamated front that would recognise the social antecedents of the problems. Although progress has been made over the last ten years, serious frailties remain in children's services and better coordination is required by all involved. The need is for less evasive clinical jargon, less rhetoric about 'children in need' and more a national programme of practical/social assessment and intervention.

THE VENEER OF THE NEW

New modes of working require new languages. For nurses, luckily, the 1970s were drenched in neologisms, the welcome mat eagerly laid out for ever more elaborate theories of nursing and its significance: this, despite any evidence that patients' problems had changed such as to warrant new descriptions, categories or interventions. But, of course, the changes had less to do with patients and more about accommodating professional interests and ambitions. Instrumental to the 'new nurse writing' (which peaked around the early 1980s with Patricia Benner's *From Novice to Expert* (1984)) were so-called post-modernist influences (see Introduction and Ch. 3) and particularly the writings of Michel Foucault (1971) who fashioned a view of language – discourse – from which, he argued, all concepts of reality stem: from now on, language determines 'reality' and defines how power is disseminated. This found its mark with mental health thinkers keen to dissolve psychiatric diagnosis and psychiatrists as 'first among equals'.

A 'postmodern turn' entered the language announcing the end of history and other grand explanations such as Marxism. People talked of 'paradigm shifts', uncertainty was in the air and even the National Health Service became subject to scrutiny and reform. Times of crises invoke 'the past' as idyllic, less encumbered with problems and criticisms. We like to imagine that, in past times, things were clearer, better financed and more liberal. We fondly recall that dissenting, aggressive patients responded positively to open systems of care, better medication and changing attitudes to mental illness. But the fact is, considerable subterfuge surrounded the changes and 'improvements' of the past. For example, pioneering open door policies were made possible by a series of camouflages. Bickford (1955), for one, sneered at these policies with their provision of refractory or 'back wards' designed to house recalcitrant patients who would otherwise have absconded and thus spoiled the party. This worked for a while; however, the run-down and imminent closure of the hospitals led to patient and public vulnerability and, gradually, public safety (and social control) re-established themselves. Unsurprisingly, concepts of dangerousness and its containment again came to the fore although newish terms would hide the custodialism they brought in their wake.

One early definition of challenging behaviour (Blunden & Allen 1987) stipulated that the challenge was to the provision of services; challenging behaviour was not an intrinsic problem of individuals. However, such superficially attractive definitions smacked of ambivalence and, in fact, challenging behaviour quickly became an additional instrument of social inference in an area already riddled with labels and jargon. Yet it is more than a label: in real terms, it justifies segregating people; it enables psychiatric nurses to dissociate from custodialism while moving their discipline, in their own eyes, towards higher professional standing. These manipulations of language substantiate Foucault's point that power is mediated by language and most effectively at local levels. So that, although typically conceived as monolithic, the NHS is as powerful in its subsidiary parts as it is at its centre – as the recent failures of particular trusts show. Pity the poor administrators with their absurd 'science of management' degrees, endlessly trying to bring doctors and nurses to heel via 'management speak' – health care delivery system, outsourced, putting stuff on the table, keeping people in the loop, performance indicators, thinking out of the box, touching base offline – ad nauseam.

KING OF THE DECEPTIONS

For psychiatric nurses, however, the king of deceptions has to be 'person-centred care' (Rogers 1967). Rogers had advocated an approach composed of empathy, non-judgementalism and unconditional positive regard. Although it provided for a humane engagement with patients, and was overwhelmingly endorsed by British nurses, it provided little guidance in respect of the majority of patients encountered in psychiatric nursing. Essentially a counselling response, it seemed ideal for dealing with problems of low esteem, social and personal adjustment but not psychosis. That being so, the acceptance of Rogerianism by psychiatric nurses constituted a false consciousness because it sidelined the awkward business of theorising about and non-medically managing psychotic patients. Protestations of empathy and non-judgementalism provided sensitive (and permissive) responses to patients overall (although few of those embracing Rogerianism disowned their allegiance to medical constructs) but they obscured mounting apprehensions about 'dangerousness' and the return of custodialism under different guises. But it was precisely these 'different guises', for example the jargon of challenging behaviour with its subtext of 'time out' rooms, 'medication management' and 'intensive care', that constituted the displacement by which nurses obfuscated the gaoler ethic.

IMPOSING CATEGORIES

Imposing a category such as 'challenging behaviour' between someone's behaviour and professional responses to it dilutes the possibility of more honest reactions. Collectively, professionals always put the idea of 'caring agency' behind their actions but this is as much to do with self-regard as it is with actual care. I imagine that challenging behaviour nurses *intend* to deliver humane and competent care: this is true of psychiatric nurses generally. Yet as Grant (1999) points out, failure to examine the restrictive features of organisations within which care occurs exposes nurses to charges of naïvety.

Throughout history, custodial regimes rarely fulfil their stated intentions of therapeutic benevolence or guarding patients' rights and wellbeing (Martin 1984). However much they try, the kind of self-scrutiny needed to do this becomes unlikely, so adrift is the custodial impulse from psychological or sociological critique.

This is not to deny that some people need secure, controlled care: rather is it to face this need honestly so as to better address the problems that go with the territory. For example, psychiatric nurses have always faced the question of how to respond when patients reject treatment. The Mental Health Act helps with this by allowing concepts of what patients 'want' to be adjusted to what they 'need'. Nurses have unerringly applied these legal twists and continue to do so. Patients who refuse are accorded the euphemism 'non-compliant' which obviates the need to take refusals as evidence of discomfort or the desire to preserve wellbeing. Because euphemisms, by their nature, serve particular circumstances and intentions, however, they quickly outlive their usefulness. So it was with 'non-compliance'; when its conformist, deferential nature became recognised it was quickly altered to 'concordance'. Whether or which, institutional psychiatry has never resolved its dual function of caring and policing. Now that mental hospitals are virtually gone, the policing function is recalibrated within the social custodialism of at-risk registers, secure facilities, risk assessments and a raft of government proposals aimed at extending compulsory treatment to patients in the community.

Against a background of yet another inquiry into the workings of forensic care (Fallon et al 1999), a former government advisor on the topic (Rowden 1998) has declared that state hospitals are woefully outdated. In addition, Aiyebusi (1998, p. 51), a forensic nursing consultant at Ashworth Special Hospital, has chronicled the 'in-house rebellion' and 'ongoing conflict' which is characteristic of forensic services, something to which I also drew attention (Clarke 1997). Of course, as Aiyebusi asserts, there exists the need to contain dangerousness. But utilising a 'new and improved' language to suggest that present-day responses are somehow more novel or refined is silly. Certainly, forensic units offer more than their predecessors; this is because, in the asylum days, we were pretty ignorant whereas, today, nurses appreciate the need for psychological interventions and are knowledgeable about them. However, offensive behaviour should be dealt with dispassionately, avoiding the psychologising which too often tries to mediate between asocial behaviour and individual responsibility. Slevin (2004) suggests that we operationalise behaviours so as to work directly with the individuals concerned and their rehabilitation. The point is that dressing custodialism with euphemisms and doubtful 'therapies' is hypocritical. If we accept that some socially objectionable behaviours, even if driven by psychological disorder, warrant custody then we should evolve structures that avoid psychologising about what are practical problems of rehabilitation inside gaoler systems.

CODA: SOME EXAMPLES

Psychiatric nursing texts have not been immune to euphemistic extravagance. Carson & Arnold (1996), for example, enthral readers with a verbal facility nowadays all too common. Employing a metaphor of 'journey', I have provided translations of some of their chapters.

- The wisdom of past travellers
- A history of mental health nursing
- Highways for the journey
- The mental health system
- Getting to know the traveller
- Mental health assessment
- Travellers from many lands
- The impact of culture

Of course, it seems right to replace the hard language of geriatrics or dementia with more user-friendly terms and, undoubtedly, the person-centred phraseology of the late Tom Kitwood (1992) actually improved practice. Difficulties arise when matters cease to be about improving care as of bolstering the writer's reputation as innovator or groundbreaker. In other cases, euphemisms may simply be about softening the blow of less agreeable aspects of care. The writer John Leo (2000) lists the creativity behind the presentation of hospital medical bills to patients:

> *"Disposable mucus recovery systems*
> *Kleenex*
> *Thermal therapy*
> *Icebags*
> *Oral administration fee*
> *Handing patients their medication"*

Leo (2000) also tells us that, in Kansas City, there is now a 'compassion zone' for homeless people which designates other areas as compassion free and thus no-go areas for vagrants. In Ireland, those whom we describe as 'learning disabled' have 'intellectual difficulties' and the problem seems to be finding a description that will stick. This has a long pedigree, from the disturbing 'idiot', 'imbecile' and 'cretin' which preceded the 1930 Mental Health Act to the even harsher 'subnormality' and 'severe subnormality' of the 1959 legislation. Are today's descriptions of people as 'special' or 'special needs' less insulting? Probably, but language mutations are an enduring feature of communication. Lavatory, for example, becomes toilet, then bathroom, then WC, then rest room. Moving on to an even more intimate plane, observe how urinate can be piss, pee, piddle, wee-wee or number ones, 'just off to visit the little boys' room' or 'powder one's nose'. In case you think I am just making this up, here are Brown & Crawford (1999, p. 42) quoting from the *International Classification of Nursing Practice* (International Council of Nurses 1996) entry for water:

> *"Water is a nursing phenomena pertaining to the physical environment with the following specific characteristics: a colourless transparent odourless, tasteless liquid compound of oxygen and hydrogen found in seas, lakes, rivers and underground and necessary for the survival of individuals. [original punctuation]"*

No comment. In the world of espionage, to assassinate is to 'terminate with extreme prejudice', in business, sacking people is 'downsizing' and when the innocent are killed in war they become 'collateral damage'.

Nurses are, therefore, not unique in wanting to make their thoughts and activities more accessible to the wider community or to themselves. We dread being seen as gaolers, doing society's dirty work of locking up psychiatric patients. But has there ever been a compulsorily detained patient who was *not* socially disruptive? And if it doesn't fall to psychiatry's practitioners to deal with this, to whom else can society turn? The fact is that, pragmatically, it turns elsewhere anyway and prisons are often the only haven available for mentally ill offenders. Perhaps this is as it should be, especially if prison psychiatry is up to scratch. It at least has the virtue of honesty. Of course, non-offenders cannot be sent to prison even if we do incarcerate them in psychiatric centres with relative ease when needed. We should not be too shy about this; acknowledging the gaoler role would bring more honesty to institutional relationships and shift the emphasis onto the legality of what happens to patients.

References

Aiyebusi A 1998 Forensic nursing is based on the flawed premise that care and custody can be combined. Nursing Times 94(8):51

Benner P 1984 From novice to expert. Addison-Wesley, California

Bickford J A R 1955 The forgotten patient. Lancet, October 29th, pp. 917–918

Blunden R, Allen D 1987 Facing the challenge: an ordinary life for people with learning difficulties and challenging behaviour. King's Fund Paper No. 74. King's Fund Centre, London

Brown B, Crawford P 1999 Putting the debate on nursing language in context. Nursing Standard 22(14):41–43

Carson V B, Arnold E N 1996 Mental health nursing: the nurse–patient journey. WB Saunders, London

Clark A 1993 Diaries. Weidenfeld & Nicolson, London

Clarke L 1997 Participant observation in a secure unit: care, conflict and control. Nursing Times Research 1:431–440

Concise Oxford English Dictionary 1977 Oxford University Press, Oxford

Fallon P, Bluglass R, Edwards B, Daniels G 1999 Report of the Committee of Inquiry into the Personality Disorder Unit, Ashworth Special Hospital. The Stationery Office, London

Foucault M 1971 Madness and civilization. Tavistock, London

Gates B 1997 Helping people towards independence. In: Gates B (ed.) Learning disabilities. Churchill Livingstone, London, pp. 135–148

Glenmullen J 2005 Experts debunk DSM. Online. Available: http://www.cchr.org/index.cfm/6519

Grant A 1999 Clinical supervision activity amongst mental health nurses: a critical organizational ethnography. Unpublished PhD thesis. University of Brighton, Brighton

International Council of Nurses 1996 The international classification for nursing practice: the alpha version. International Council of Nurses, Geneva

Kitwood T 1992 Person to person: a guide to the care of those with failing mental powers. Gale Centre Publications, Loughton

Kubrick S 1964 Dr. Strangelove: or how I learned to stop worrying and love the bomb. Columbia Pictures, California

Kushlick A 1996 Providing supportive services. The Open University Press, Milton Keynes

Leo J 2000 Incorrect thoughts: notes on our wayward culture. Transaction Publishers, New Jersey

Martin J P 1984 Hospitals in trouble. Blackwell, Oxford

Mitchell R 2003 Ideological reflections on the DSM-IV-R (or pay no attention to the man behind the curtain, Dorothy!). Child and Youth Care Forum 32(5):281–298

Mount F 1997 This feeble, phoney war on child abuse. The Sunday Times, News Review Section, November 23rd, p. 4

Mullan B 1999 R D Laing: a personal view. Duckworth, London

Rogers C 1967 On becoming a person. Constable, London

Rose J, Walker S 1997 Home for people with challenging behaviours. Nursing Times 93:54–55

Rowden R 1998 Shut that door. Nursing Times 94(4):14–15

Slevin E 2004 Learning disabilities: a survey of community nurses for people with prevalence of challenging behaviour and contact demands. Journal of Clinical Nursing 13(5):571–579

Bibliography

Neaman J S, Silver C G 1983 Kind words: a thesaurus of euphemisms. Facts on File, New York

Newbrook C 2005 Ducks in a row: the definitive guide to office English. Short Books, London

Rawson H 1981 A dictionary of euphemisms and other doubletalk. Crown Publishers, New York

20

Virtual insanity: imag(in)ing illness in brain scans of schizophrenic people

Dave, I don't understand why you're doing this to me. You're destroying my mind. Don't you understand? I will become nothing

(Computer HAL 9000)

MACHINES

The late film director Stanley Kubrick was fascinated by the possibilities of artificial intelligence (AI) and was slated to make a movie about it. When he died, Steven Spielberg (2001) took over, producing his own version. Called *AI*, it lacked Kubrick's superficial profundity but displayed his fascination with disembodied intelligence and the caprice of machines. In Kubrick's earlier film, *2001: A Space Odyssey* (1968), human nature is transcended (by machines), the astronauts occupying subsidiary, characterless roles with the spaceship's computer (HAL 9000) displaying a 'humanity' that embraces apprehension, cynicism, slyness, humour, aggression and fear. Disappointed with the astronauts' performance, HAL tries to take over the spaceship while it journeys towards Jupiter. On discovering this, the astronauts begin dismantling HAL by removing 'his' microchips. HAL's cry: 'I will become nothing' implies that, somehow, consciousness has been implanted into 'his' hardware, into who 'he' is. More recent films, for example *I, Robot* (Proyas 2004), also depict robotic intelligence initially programmed to operate compliantly but becoming more autonomous (and aggressive) over time. Usually the machines turn into killers, either because so programmed by a 'mad scientist' or, intriguingly, some kind of micro-chip mutation incites them to self-awareness, whereby they engage in complex, aggressive behaviours as if driven by something analogous to human thinking.

Not so ourselves of course; when it comes to us we employ concepts of 'the self' with unwavering conviction. Self-esteem, determination, worth, regard, all of these comprise a self-evident selfhood and 'I' trips off the tongue more easily than any other word. Indeed, it is the ability to begin sentences with 'I' that makes us unique. So much so that from time immemorial we have striven to show what constitutes this 'I' and where it resides. Does it, robotic fashion, inhabit a hardware system – the brain – or does it lie within a much less discernible domain – the mind? Perhaps, like other species, we are composed of mere bundles of behaviours, set in our courses by little more than habituation to stimulus–response systems.

THE GHOST IN THE MACHINE

Gilbert Ryle believed that concepts of selfhood were problematic; in his book *The Concept of Mind* (1949) he used a 'ghost in the machine' motif to reject the Cartesian principle that the brain co-exists with a 'soul'. This is the so-called dualist position which holds that the material and immaterial are in check, neither accounting for the other. In modern parlance, the word soul is replaced with mind, the equation now constituting the 'body–mind problem'. Ryle's solution to the problem was to abolish the mind, to discard thinking and feeling as necessary intermediaries between the organism's environmental stimuli and its responses (behaviours). According to Ryle, to assume that between each given stimulus and its response lies a consciousness – a self – that governs the whole process is mistaken. Rather, ideas are ways of behaving, part of the complex of responding; they are not an integrated 'I' but, instead, the cognitive component of responses. Paraphrasing Descartes' 'I think therefore I am' to 'There are thoughts therefore there are thoughts' will help us understand what is meant here. However, we *like* to infer 'I'; we dislike the unpalatability of ourselves as mere bundles of conditioned responses. Thus our fascination with machines that 'think'; we are simply not used to seeing things any other way.

PROBLEMS

Collapsing thought into behaviour is problematic though. For instance, that I need to be observing my behaviour so as to have an awareness of something seems doubtful. For instance, can't I experience happiness without having behavioural indicators that suggest it? Conversely, might I not feel deeply ashamed of something when in others' company but not show it? In the latter instance, if I am not behaving 'something' then it must be asked what is the 'something' I am not behaving? And if this something requires some kind of existence, then why not call it mind? In an intriguing contribution to the mind/brain problem Nobel Prize winning physicist Sir Arthur Eccles (1982a, 1982b) asks how humans can have an 'awareness of awareness' and he argues that if such awareness(es) could run to infinity there would not be enough brain to contain them! The implausibility of this is not helped by the curious difficulty of mounting an argument against it.

Another, less abstract, take on the mind–brain problem is the James–Lange Theory. Proposed separately (by psychologists William James and Carl Lange) James (1896, pp. 375–376) describes it thus:

> *"My theory is that the bodily changes follow the perception of the exciting fact, and that our feeling of the changes, as they occur, is the emotion. Common sense says we are frightened and run; we are insulted, are angry, and strike. This order of sequence is incorrect … and that the more rational statement is that we feel sorry because we cry, angry because we strike, afraid because we tremble."*

James sensed the paradox in this and suspected that people would intuitively reject it. What it proposes *is* perplexing: that my perception of an event – be it threatening or tragic – will excite my autonomic nervous system and that it is this that makes me fear. If I am frightened and run, my running creates a loop within my central nervous system whereby 'because I am running, I must be afraid'. I suppose it's not unlike eating a sandwich and remarking: 'Oh, I must have been hungry'. Cognitive behavioural therapists would support the loop element because of its relevance to treating anxiety, especially panic. They would try to break the loop by helping patients to deploy cognitive strategies that eliminate the debilitating aspects of their responses. So, even when we construe thought as behaviour, patients can be helped to 'instruct' noxious thinking either to stop or to convert to pleasantness. This too suggests an 'I' of sorts, a self force that can opt for some thoughts over others, something that smacks less of thought as action and more about aspiration, need or desire.

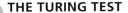

THE TURING TEST

Developed by a contemporary of Ryle's, this test states that if a computer can make experts believe that it is thinking then it is thinking! John Searle's (1983) response to the Turing test still suffices. He posits a Chinese Room inside which someone has an instruction book instructing him or her how to respond. Chinese language symbols are passed into the room and the job of the person with the instruction book is to pass back appropriate symbols in turn. This person doesn't know Chinese but this is irrelevant since the book contains all the instructions he needs. Searle's point is that you might convince a Chinese speaker (outside the room) that you know the language when actually you don't. In fact, given the nature of computerised instructions, no one inside the Chinese room – i.e. the computer – need know the language, not even the instruction book! What this experiment shows is that software – which is itself ignorant – can give rise to phenomena which appear to comprehend but which have simply been programmed to look that way. Yet it is not thinking. For Searle, the hardware is the thing and he sees biology as giving rise to consciousness not as a 'new' or separate entity but as a higher level function of itself. What researchers have done is confuse 'how' with 'that'. In other words, that we do not yet know *how* biology produces consciousness is no barrier to believing that it does.

PAIRED REALITIES

D. H. Lawrence would have disagreed. Lawrence once said that water was two molecules of hydrogen and one of oxygen and *something else*, the something else that makes it wet. For Searle, and scientists generally, water's external property, its wetness, is consistent with the molecular bonding that makes this property up and that this is inexplicable: water is what it is. It hardly surprises, given the evidence base of this supposition, that most scientists are disinclined to dabble in questions about consciousness! This reluctance underpins their conviction that science deals best with objectivity and what remains is cast into a subjective, irretrievable limbo. Such reasoning fuels the supposed explanatory superiority of the scientific (material) over the impressionistic (immaterial) but in passing playing down the difficulties that this throws up. The difficulty becomes clear in Hanfling's (1978) recount of Eddington's (1935) 'two tables' discourse:

> *"One of them had been familiar to me from earlier years. It is a commonplace object of that environment which I call the world.*

How shall I describe it? It has extension; it is comparatively permanent; it is coloured; above all it is substantial ... Table no. 2 is my scientific table. My scientific table is mostly emptiness. Sparsely scattered in that emptiness are numerous electrical charges rushing about with great speed; but their combined bulk amounts to less than a billionth of the bulk of the table itself. There is nothing substantial about my second table. It is nearly all empty space ... I need not tell you that modern physics had by delicate test and remorseless logic assured me that my second scientific table is the only one which is really there."

Whew! Eddington's discourse falls squarely within a 'science has shown' mode of argument. There is an 'it goes without saying' quality to it; 'I need not tell you', he states, of the 'remorseless logic' by which such conclusions are reached. Two consequences flow from this: one is the 'hidden persuasiveness', the proselytising, which often informs 'scientific discourse', a 'we are almost there' tendency which is often present. Second are the over-estimates of what actually has been shown. Of particular relevance are claims about mental illness as a product of brain pathology with a concomitant playing down of the role of experience. This representation of the mind/brain problem in clinical terms has become a flashpoint for many psychiatric nurses. As nursing is practice based, debates have naturally crystallised around such things as interventions, styles of research, patients' narratives, and the importance of pharmacology. For example, the issue of psychiatric nurse prescribing has tended to band nurses around either an experiential position which underpins a non-prescribing stance or a brain pathology standpoint which, generally, favours the opposite.

CONSTRUCTS OF ILLNESS

Locating experience within nervous systems is never easy. Constructs of illness depend upon representations but, unlike Eddington's scientific table, they also require depth and substance. X-ray imagery, for instance, is basic to the practice of medicine. X-rays have made our lives safe in all sorts of ways, from denoting pathology to detecting the murderous intent of ticking devices in suitcases. While indispensable, X-rays hardly match the safety of MRI (magnetic resonance imaging) nor the in-depth, three-dimensional inspections of the CAT (computed axial tomography) scan and we are now in a position to 'see' far more than we could even half a generation ago. But what exactly do we see? Several years ago

I watched transfixed as a medical doctor employed by the (then) National Coal Board strove to play down, during a television interview, the compensation claims of coal miners with pneumoconiosis. Asked whether those with greater degrees of the disease should receive greater compensation, he replied that, indeed, pneumoconiosis was not a disease: 'rather was it', he said, 'a radiological picture'. Thus, when required, was the distinction between illness and artefact declared a matter of interpretation. Rather than utilise the X-ray pictures to bolster the miners' claims, their pathology was trivialised, its connections to their experience excluded.

In psychiatry, one comes across this quite a lot: interpreting meaningful links between artefacts and 'underlying illnesses' albeit aiming towards opposite conclusions to that of the Coal Board. In psychiatric research, the tendency is to seize upon any CAT scan or PET (positron emission tomography) scan imagery that suggests differences between schizophrenic people and samples chosen from normal populations. In effect, it is claimed that PET scan pictures show the very disease itself. Such machines, says Krueger (1991, p. 4), provide 'a means of visualising thought'. According to Stafford (1996, p. 24):

> *"Computer simulation of the brain's interconnected nerve cells provides neuroscientists and cognitive psychologists with literal insights into the dynamic processes by which the mind thinks, senses, feels."*

Cairns-Smith (1996, p. 155) adds that 'with such machines one can almost watch someone thinking'. Yet what this overlooks is that the word schizophrenia describes mental conditions whose boundaries, putting it mildly, are vaguely defined. Yet this is thrashed by PET scan readings supposedly representing the inner workings of something that has descriptive value only. Contrasting the enthusiasm of psychiatric bio-medicalists with those working in physical medicine yields a more temperate approach. Hampton (1992), for example, states that the ECG (electrocardiogram) 'is not an end in itself' and that 'interpreting [it] is only a small part of making a cardiac diagnosis'. Whereas, in psychiatry, technological etchings from PET and CAT scans are unhesitatingly heralded as manifestations of psychological illness.

HUMAN LITHOGRAPHS

Such claims diminish the contribution of non-experts, regrettably so because the views of service users are vital to discussions about schizophrenia. Such narratives do not rule out schizophrenia as a disease, but they do contrast medical perspectives with the experience of it. For one can know just about everything there is to know about schizophrenia as a disease 'without being able to understand a single schizophrenic' (Laing 1960, p. 33). Spiralling down into reductive analysis enhances medical precision about mental illness but diminishes psychological and social correlates. Of course, physicians will reply that disease is their business and why should befriending or even knowing patients be part of the job? Strictly speaking this is true but, taken to its limits, it reduces medicine to a medieval dispensing of potions. A leading physical treatment psychiatrist, William Sargant, reflected this when he anticipated a psychiatry that would diagnose depression, treat it with electricity on an out-patient basis before sending the patient home: a bit like setting a broken bone and without all that tiresome business of history taking and psychologising.

ILLNESS

The medical/nursing take on schizophrenia rests on propositions of defect rather than difference. For example, it would be surprising were PET scans on brain blood flow correlated with, say, attitudes towards ethnic minorities. Were this to happen, it's unlikely that racism would be categorised as mental defect: as a rule, this is not how we act towards racists. We could psychologise about them at length and no doubt some do. In general, however, though racists exult in dangerous, irrational, perverse and deluded beliefs, we rightly judge them from moral, not psychiatric, standpoints. Not so schizophrenic beliefs which are perceived as so odd that the only explanation that makes any sense is illness. Yet to assert that schizophrenia manifests itself in PET scan pictures is to exaggerate the power of scans. If we are reluctant to correlate PET scan pictures with racism, then why the ease with which we do it with schizophrenia? And it is insufficient to argue that racism is culturally/historically defined as anti-social whereas schizophrenia is not since, if so, how come? In fact, considerable social construction, independent of medical evidence, attends the formation of beliefs about schizophrenia. LeVay's (1991) paper makes this clear. In a controlled study, LeVay, who is gay and a gay rights campaigner, located brain tissue that differed in respect of sexual orientation in males. It led him to conclude that sexual orientation was at least 50% biological in origin. Aware of the political ramifications of this, LeVay nevertheless argued the advantages of homosexuality as biologically driven since this killed the idea of *choosing* to be gay – i.e. gays as abnormal heterosexuals, an established tenet of homophobic thought. Yet LeVay was also sensitive about centralising biology because this might spark the usual drive to 'cure the condition' by physical methods.

The question for us, though, is allowing that brain differences exist between gays and straights, does this enable us to label gays as 'abnormal' or 'ill'? Or would we incline towards describing both groups as different? What LeVay shows is that diagnoses of schizophrenia depend on *prior* beliefs about what counts as normal/abnormal behaviour. Such diagnoses rest on twin assumptions: first, statistical inferences – what would the world look like if 42% of its inhabitants were schizophrenic? It's difficult to say but, comparatively speaking, schizophrenics would be in a more ascendant position! As it is, the 1% incidence of schizophrenia is the lynchpin in its conception as illness. Second, because homosexuality is now considered normal we can fairly ask: what price from LeVay's findings on biology? The answer is none since 'gay as mental illness' is no longer feasible. The point is that it was always a social construction and while biology can influence how we see things it is not a determining factor.

NO TWISTED THOUGHT WITHOUT A TWISTED MOLECULE (GERARD 1956)

Asserting the psychiatric significance of PET scan pictures has nevertheless become a vibrant activity within some psychiatric nursing circles. For example, Professor Gournay (1996, p. 8) states:

> *"There are now numerous studies that report structural abnormalities in the brains of people with schizophrenia."*

True. However, there are equal numbers of studies which demonstrate similar abnormalities in non-schizophrenic brains as well (Dawson 1997). In a sustained critique of the field, Raeburn (2005, p. 70) had his own brain scanned by a noted psychiatric researcher: the scan showed no abnormalities nor, given the wide variability in normal brain structure and function, was it likely to. Raeburn considered that his researcher:

> *"would not have been able to conclude much specifically about how my brain differs from those of other people."*

In other words, 'mechanical images' reveal little except in cases where there are specific brain lesions. In the case of schizophrenia they may occasionally reveal abnormalities which are not exclusive to schizophrenia or, indeed, may be as much an *outcome* of mental distress as its *cause*.

Professor Gournay (1996, p. 8) further states:

> "*Because these techniques [PET scans] allow very precise measurement, researchers are now able to carry out careful experiments, looking at individuals over the course of time or comparing individuals with schizophrenia with control populations.*"

Note the juxtaposition of '*very precise* measurement', '*careful* experiments' and '*individuals with schizophrenia*'. Here is the 'science has shown' gambit again, the belief that these pictures possess explanatory power when they are merely descriptive. As Jenner et al (1993, p. 49) point out, such statements:

> "*show very clearly how powerful technical language is and how dangerously we manipulate words in order to settle questions that in reality are still waiting for a proper solution.*"

There is nothing new in this; deploying science to solve problems in living is as old as the hills.

THE PAST REPEATS ITSELF

Forty years ago, Hans Eysenck (1967) made connections between nervous systems and human behaviour in areas of intelligence and its measurement. His mentor, Sir Cyril Burt, fabricated data so as to forge links between heredity and, this time, poor academic progress (Hearnshaw 1979). In both instances the ethical and human consequences were clear: in Burt's case, many of the nation's children were consigned to an inappropriate 'education' following poor performance on the 11-plus examination. Later still, generations of learning disabilities children were denied a balanced assessment of their abilities because of the IQ testing which Eysenck, among others, had championed. Believing that such tests set 'the ceiling' on children's capacities, psychologists' reports became benchmarks for pessimism and therapeutic laziness. Thus did externally contrived 'scans' of children's intelligence consign those not 'making the grade' to a second tier education or to learning disability, both categories precluding meaningful interventions to help them. Much of this resulted from the therapeutic euphoria accompanying 'new findings', in this case psychometrics, and the belief that what they measured was innate, fixed, biological, irredeemable. We can learn from this by pondering the ethics of supposing that anatomical structure or biochemistry are causal factors in human behaviour.

VIRTUAL TREATMENTS

Yet researchers enthuse about the new technology; they eagerly anticipate computer mapping of brain function and the construction of virtual worlds via computer simulation. Riva & Vincelli (2001) describe how virtual reality programmes enhance the efficacy of psychotherapy by inducing in clients an awareness of being skilled at solving problems in their virtual state. Sherman & Judkin (1993) have explored the therapeutic applications of this and believe that simulated treatments for phobias are feasible. Wooley (1992, p. 280) agrees:

> "*Applications of virtual reality to the treatment of fears and phobias and stress reactions, are the likeliest first targets for medical researchers.*"

Virtual reality's most likely enthusiasts, states Wooley, will be cognitive behaviour therapists who will actually find it irresistible. However, ethics again raises its head. Is it ethical to embark on research which attempts to supply subjects with alternative virtual worlds? For instance, considering the nature of addiction, how would recipients of virtual realities be able, following habituation, to distinguish real from unreal? And what about the ethical implications of withdrawing 'virtuality' if patients preferred it to their illness state? If people entered virtual realities as a calming exercise wouldn't it be cruel to bring them out of these involuntarily? And if they remained within their virtual systems, wouldn't this vandalise who they *really* are: a case of virtual murder?

These things are not far fetched: audio-relaxation tapes, for instance, are well established. In 1998, White reported that 50% of patients, logging on to a specially designed CD-ROM obtained reductions in anxiety symptoms. Currently, some psychiatric units invite patients to enter 'Snoezelen rooms' (Long & Haigh 1992) kitted out with technology-induced calming mechanisms (music, altered imagery, fibre optics). Extending this to metaphor, might we one day envisage corporate virtual systems where patients share an intersubjective cyberspace; virtual nursing homes, perhaps, where placid 'realities', derived from 'reality orientation' principles, re-focus debilitated nervous systems, in effect prompting people to forget that they have forgotten.

What virtual technology does is concretise symbolic constructions, making them potentially applicable. But usefulness is questionable where the technology brings loss of status or dignity for those involved. Far from helping psychotic people, virtual realities might induce dehumanisation, not in the usual senses of labelling and stigmatising, but in a post-Turingian, post-Kubrickian sense of fusing machines and biology as though of equal merit, substituting artificial experience for faltering brain–bodies. In the movie *Dr. Strangelove: or How I Learned to Stop Worrying and Love the Bomb*, Stanley Kubrick (1964) pushed the idea to its limits with malevolent, warmongering Dr. Strangelove advocating nuclear holocaust while agonisingly trying to prevent his right arm from making Nazi salutes. The arm – be it bionic or sentient – operates independently of Strangelove and at one point it even tries to strangle him. The possibilities of such things draw near; for example, marrying mechanics to cerebral biology so as to regenerate post-traumatic limb movement is now commonplace. Whether such machinations will one day transmit more than motor impulses, whether they will ultimately be able to propel neuro-conscious 'particles' into the body, following transplantation, or without the body, is unlikely.

LEAVING THE BODY OUT

With PET scan imaging we are in danger of losing our minds. These machines lengthen the distance between experiential worlds and medical discourses. With PET scans, psychiatry represents schizophrenia as a post-human condition. Says Ansell Pearson (1997, p. 124):

> "The task of the new technologies is to unblock the 'obstacle' constituted on earth by human life"

and by doing so draw us nearer to the Baudrillardian (1996) nightmare of 'thought without bodies'. Technology is science made operational by desire. However, that which is desirable is not external to technology but intrinsic to its uses: the machines' aptitudes bring about new problems but, equally, do they hint at solutions. That said, is it too rash to assume that machines might one day experience things? In human terms, this:

> "is the nub of the problem. No amount of anatomical description can actually tell you what it is like to experience."

> (Cornwell 1997, p. 62)

And if this is true for anatomy, it is certainly true for machines. However, we might like to consider here a difference between experiencing and cognition insofar as if the machine could deductively arrive at solutions, as ably as any human, could this not be construed as a kind of thinking?

BUT WHERE IS CYBERSPACE AND WHY IS IT VIRTUAL?

William Gibson (2001) said he invented the term cyberspace to describe 'consensual hallucination'; that is, a predilection to become so immersed in the media that the interpersonal life is denied. Certainly, in space and time, McLuhan's 'global village' is now among us and, for many, reality is now the Internet, texting, PET scans and MTV! As in Vietnam, as in the Balkans, wars are won and lost on the immediacy of their distilled imagery on our televisions. The television set is our alter ego, the means by which our lesser selves – be it in terms of buying or selling, diet or detox, fitness or flab – are acted out for us. In one of its manifestations, 'reality TV', we encounter the Orwellian nightmare, although these days the rats in the head cage are less cause for horror, more occasions for laughter. The 2006 *Big Brother* show bears this out, its contestants comprising someone alleged to be suicidal, a recovering anorexic, someone with Tourette's syndrome, a pre-operative transsexual and someone with body dysmorphic disorder. It led Marjorie Wallace (2006), chief executive of SANE, to liken the whole business to 'bear baiting'. She has a point: at least in the days of Bedlam one paid a penny to watch 'the lunatics'. Voyeurism is everywhere now, almost a national sport. Of course, the *Big Brother* contestants are voluntary, no one forces them into it; the shame lies with those of us who egg them on.

We are of course not unaware of the downside to this and have been for some time. The film *The Truman Show* (Weir 1998) – based on MTV's *The Real World* – showed human exploitation taken to new limits. This movie portrayed a virtual world inside a giant dome, peopled by actors, and with a single human, Truman, brought up to believe that life in the dome is real. Transmitted as a 24-hour 'soap' Truman only discovers 'reality' when the physical mechanics of the subterfuge begin to go awry. When he tries to leave, the soap's creator tells him that his invented world is better than the 'real thing' and that unhappiness awaits if he leaves. But by whose reasoning, retorts Truman, is this invented world more real? True, it is entirely anodyne, pain free, banal and rarely distressing, a place where ignorance has finally become bliss. But it is also bereft of genuine human encounter, of knowledge and true awareness of what things mean.

Similarly, in *The Matrix* (Wachowski 1999), the protagonist believes that he lives in a city, that it is sunny outside and that he has hair. But he has no hair; in fact, he hasn't anything, he is a brain suspended in a vat. On reflection, is it conceivable, as I write this, that *I* am inside a Matrix, duped in respect of my existence? Recall the Turing test and the Chinese Room, that if the computer makes us believe it is thinking then it *is* thinking. To wit, believing that I am me, when I am 'in fact' a brain hooked up to a mechanism that floats me in a vat means that 'I' am virtual and nothing more. This was Descartes' question 400 years ago, that think I, then, therefore, am I? How do I know that I'm not just a figment in the mind of an evil genius who controls the universe? Disputing this evil genius notion is difficult yet, there has to be a starting point at which reason finds manifest the truth of its ideas and Descartes is as good a place as any.

PERSON-MACHINES

Richard Dawkins (1978, p. x) states:

> *"We are robot vehicles blindly programmed to preserve the selfish molecules known as genes."*

Stove (1992) notes that socio-biologists like Dawkins carefully add that while humans carry 'selfish genes' this doesn't imply that genes are conscious: yet, says Stove:

> *"Where sociobiologists differ from other people is just that they also say, over and over again, things which imply that genes are [his emphasis] conscious purposeful agents."*

This represents extreme biological determinism where claims about 'free will' become as suspect as transcendence, spirituality or brainless psychosis. The latter are distractions, illusions that create impressions of self-fulfilment but which really just protect the genes which evolve the organism and so on. But while conceding that science informs us about the facts of cases we question whether it can determine our responses. For example, if there are biological dimensions to schizophrenia this doesn't mean that we see it exclusively as such. Judgements of value impact on how we evaluate mental illness even if this position is currently under attack from encroaching biotechnology and its representations. Particularly insidious has been the development of photographing the scars of people who self harm and depicting these as 'galleries' on Internet websites, an activity described by Louise Pembroke (2004) as 'medical pornography'. As Sander Gilman (1988, p. 48) states:

"The tradition of representing madness in the form of icons ... points towards the need by society to identify the mad absolutely. Society must be able to localise and confine the mad, if only visually, in order to create a separation between the sane and the insane."

What better actualisation of human experience – of supposed mental illness – than reification through hardwired systems which reconstitute madness in three dimensions and Technicolor. In an age where communication is fully digitalised, should we be surprised at this?

References

Ansell Pearson K 1997 Viroid life. Routledge, London

Baudrillard J 1996 The system of objects. Sage, London

Cairns-Smith A G 1996 Evolving the mind: on the nature of matter and the origins of consciousness. Cambridge University Press, Cambridge

Cornwell R J 1997 You cannot be serious. The Sunday Times Magazine, June 15th, pp. 56–62

Dawkins R 1978 The selfish gene. Paladin, London

Dawson P J 1997 A reply to Kevin Gournay's schizophrenia: a review of the contemporary literature and implications for mental health nursing theory, practice and education. Journal of Psychiatric and Mental Health Nursing 4:1–7

Eccles J 1982a The human brain and the human person. In: Eccles J (ed.) Mind and brain: the many faceted problems. Paragon Press, Washington, DC, pp. 81–98

Eccles J 1982b A critical appraisal of brain–mind theories. In: Eccles J (ed.) Mind and brain: the many faceted problems. Paragon Press, Washington, DC, pp. 239–245

Eddington A 1935 The nature of the physical world. Everyman Editions, London

Eysenck H J 1967 The biological basis of personality. Charles C Thomas, Springfield, Illinois

Gerard R W 1956 Comments: In: Cole J, Gerard R J (eds) Psychopharmacology: problems in evaluation. National Academy of Sciences, National Research Council, Washington, DC

Gibson W 2001 Neuromancer. Voyager, London

Gilman S L 1988 Diseases and representation: images of illness from madness to AIDS. Cornell University Press, London

Gournay K 1996 Schizophrenia: a review of the contemporary literature and implications for mental health nursing, theory, practice and education. Journal of Psychiatric and Mental Health Nursing 3:7–12

Hampton J R 1992 The EEG in practice, 2nd edn. Churchill Livingstone, London

Hanfling O 1978 Uses and abuses of argument. An arts foundation course: Units 2b & 9. The Open University Press, Milton Keynes

Hearnshaw L S 1979 Cyril Burt: psychologist. Hodder & Stoughton, London

James W 1896 Textbook of psychology. Macmillan, London

Jenner F A, Monteiro A C D, Zagalo-Cardoso J A et al 1993 Schizophrenia: a disease or some ways of being human. Sheffield Academic Press, Sheffield

Krueger M W 1991 Artificial reality II. Addison-Wesley, London

Kubrick S 1964 Dr. Strangelove: or how I learned to stop worrying and love the bomb. Columbia Pictures, California

Kubrick S 1968 2001: a space odyssey. Warner Brothers, California

Laing R D 1960 The voice of experience. Pantheon Books, New York

LeVay S 1991 A difference in hypothalamic structure between homosexual and heterosexual men. Science 253:1034–1037

Long A P, Haigh L 1992 How do clients benefit from Snoezelen: an exploratory study. British Journal of Occupational Therapy 53: 103–106

Pembroke L 2004 Medical pornography. Open Mind 130:12–13

Proyas A 2004 I, robot. 20th Century Fox, California

Raeburn P 2005 MRI: a window on the brain. Technology Review 108(11):70

Riva G, Vincelli F 2001 Virtual reality as an advanced imaginal system: a new experiential approach for counselling and therapy. International Journal of Action Methods: Psychodrama, Skill Training, and Role Playing, June 22nd. Online. Available: http://www.highbeam.com/doc/1G1-95765052.html

Ryle G 1949 The concept of mind. Hutchinson, London

Searle J 1983 Intentionality: an essay in the philosophy of mind. Cambridge University Press, Cambridge

Sherman B, Judkin P 1993 Glimpses of heaven, visions of hell: virtual reality and its implications. Coronet Books, London

Spielberg S 2001 AI. Warner Brothers, California

Stafford B M 1996 Good looking: essays on the virtue of images. The MIT Press, London

Stove D 1992 A new religion. Online. Available: http://www.royalinstitutephilosophy.org/articles/article.php?id=27

Wachowski A 1999 The matrix. Warner Brothers, California

Wallace M 2006 Worse than bear baiting. Daily Mail, June 1st, pp. 31–33

Weir P 1998 The Truman show. Paramount Pictures, California

White J 1998 'Stresspack': three-year follow-up of a controlled trial of self-help package for the anxiety disorders. Behavioral and Cognitive Psychotherapy 26:133–141

Wooley B 1992 Virtual worlds: a journey through hype and hyperreality. Blackwell, Oxford

Conclusion

Journey's end. Time to inquire if anything has been learnt and what, if anything, can be concluded. Were we to be observed by the proverbial 'little man from Mars' he would conclude that psychiatric nursing is in a state of flux with doubt and debate plaguing many of its activities and ambitions. We have seen that this is not true for those wanting to define the profession as a medical or quasi-medical activity or as a psychological discipline delivering cognitive behavioural therapy or its alternatives. They, arguably, possess the clearest vision of psychiatric nursing's future albeit with a loss of essence as to what psychiatric nursing is in and of itself.

Beginning with research, we discovered no particular route to evidence-based truth which accurately encompasses questions to which psychiatric nurses seek answers. Thus did succeeding chapters raise issues of ethics, legality and rights which remain unresolved because they are not susceptible to the empirical inquiries represented by randomised controlled trials. There continues to be much about psychiatric nursing that requires professional, political and ethical review as well as reform. For example, the manner by which culture, history, ethnicity and social exclusion impact on people's mental health has been shown to be of first importance and an indication of the breadth and depth of responses needed from community psychiatric nurses. Apart from the enhanced power to prescribe drugs, the lives of patients are construed by myriad political and economic forces and, indeed, even the manner by which diagnoses of mental illness are made results in part from historically determined attitudes of what counts as normal and what doesn't.

Psychiatric nurses do not spring, Athene like, into existence. They are forged by their societies into thinking about nursing in particular ways. They bring these primitive notions to the nursing academy whose role becomes the process of moulding them into more learned concepts of the profession's attitudes and obligations. We have discovered, however, just how out of kilter these intellectual concepts may be and how an ages-old problem of 'theory–practice divide' has, in fact, been exacerbated by the rush into the universities in the absence of evidence that this was sought by the broad base of practitioners.

To an extent, this academic ascendancy has given rise to preoccupations – we looked at continental philosophising, extended vocabularies of jargon, curricular flights of fancy, pretensions to scientific research status – which have disastrously led to a neglect of more pressing issues of standards of daily care, ethical status and protection of patients' welfare and rights. There is now emerging a palpable sense which seeks to re-inculcate in psychiatric nurses more practical aspects of care, what are called basic or foundational skills. This, however, competes with higher aspirations to prescribe medicines and perform discrete psychological therapies. Psychiatric nursing is a broad spectrum activity and we must content ourselves with its divisions and varying orientations. Yet one cannot but reflect, amid all of this, that something essential – what defines psychiatric *nursing* – is missing. Further, given the ethical background that fuels many of the issues in these pages, especially as directly related to patients, there yet seems to be room – above considerations of techniques, therapies, models or treatments – for the application of ordinary decency to people in the wider contexts of their humanity.

Index

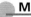

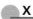